Exotic Animal Training and Learning

Guest Editor

BARBARA HEIDENREICH

VETERINARY CLINICS
OF NORTH AMERICA:
EXOTIC ANIMAL PRACTICE

www.vetexotic.theclinics.com

Consulting Editor
AGNES E. RUPLEY, DVM, Dipl. ABVP–Avian

September 2012 • Volume 15 • Number 3

SAUNDERS an imprint of ELSEVIER, Inc.

W.B. SAUNDERS COMPANY
A Division of Elsevier Inc.
1600 John F. Kennedy Boulevard ● Suite 1800 ● Philadelphia, Pennsylvania 19103-2899
http://www.vetexotic.theclinics.com

VETERINARY CLINICS OF NORTH AMERICA: EXOTIC ANIMAL PRACTICE Volume 15, Number 3
September 2012 ISSN 1094-9194, ISBN-13: 978-1-4557-4968-3

Editor: John Vassallo; j.vassallo@elsevier.com
Development Editor: Teia Stone

Veterinary Clinics of North America: Exotic Animal Practice (ISSN 1094-9194) is published in January, May, and September by Elsevier, Inc., 360 Park Avenue South, New York, NY 10010-1710. Subscription prices are $229.00 per year for US individuals, $367.00 per year for US institutions, $117.00 per year for US students and residents, $273.00 per year for Canadian individuals, $433.00 per year for Canadian institutions, $308.00 per year for international individuals, $433.00 per year for international institutions and $150.00 per year for Canadian and foreign students/ residents. To receive student/resident rate, orders must be accompanied by name of affiliated institution, date of term, and the *signature* of program/residency coordinator on institution letterhead. Orders will be billed at individual rate until proof of status is received. Foreign air speed delivery is included in all *Clinics* subscription prices. All prices are subject to change without notice. **POSTMASTER:** Send address changes to *Veterinary Clinics of North America: Exotic Animal Practice*, Elsevier Health Sciences Division, Subscription Customer Service, 3251 Riverport Lane, Maryland Heights, MO 63043. **Customer Service: Telephone: 1-800-654-2452** (U.S. and Canada); **1-314-447-8871** (outside U.S. and Canada). **Fax: 1-314-447-8029. E-mail:journalscustomerservice-usa@elsevier.com** (for print support); **journalsonlinesupport-usa@elsevier.com** (for online support).

Reprints. For copies of 100 or more of articles in this publication, please contact the Commercial Reprints Department, Elsevier Inc., 360 Park Avenue South, New York, New York 10010-1710. Tel.: (212)-633-3813; Fax: (212)-633-1935; E-mail: reprints@elsevier.com.

Veterinary Clinics of North America: Exotic Animal Practice is covered in *MEDLINE/PubMed (Index Medicus).*

Printed and bound by CPI Group (UK) Ltd, Croydon, CR0 4YY

Transferred to digital print 2012

Contributors

CONSULTING EDITOR

AGNES E. RUPLEY, DVM
Diplomate, American Board of Veterinary Practitioners–Avian Practice; Director and Chief Veterinarian, All Pets Medical & Laser Surgical Center, College Station, Texas

GUEST EDITOR

BARBARA HEIDENREICH, BS(Zoology)
Good Bird Inc, Austin, Texas

AUTHORS

LAUREN AUGUSTINE, BA
Animal Keeper, Department of Animal Programs, Smithsonian's National Zoological Park, Washington, DC

SABRINA I.C.A. BRANDO, BSc
AnimalConcepts, Lelystad, The Netherlands

SUSAN A. BROWN, DVM
The Behavior Connection, North Aurora, Illinois

ELLEN K. COOK, DVM
Cicero Veterinary Clinic, Cicero, Indiana

ALLISON L. CORWIN, BS(Biology)
Animals, Science and the Environment, Disney's The Seas®, Lake Buena Vista, Florida

PARVENE FARHOODY, MA
PhD Candidate, Learning Processes and Behavior Analysis, and Adjunct Professor, Department of Psychology, Queens College, Graduate Center of the City University of New York, Flushing, New York

BARBARA HEIDENREICH, BS(Zoology)
Good Bird Inc, Austin, Texas

HEIDI HELLMUTH, BS
Curator, Department of Animal Programs, Smithsonian's National Zoological Park, Washington, DC

KATHARINE HOPE, DVM
Associate Veterinarian, Department of Animal Health, Smithsonian's National Zoological Park, Washington, DC

GAIL LAULE, MA
Active Environments, Inc, Lompoc, California

SARA MATTISON, BS, MMin
Staff Biologist, Point Defiance Zoo & Aquarium, Tacoma, Washington

REBECCA K. O'CONNOR
Animal Behavior Consultant, Banning, California

KEN RAMIREZ
Shedd Aquarium, Chicago, Illinois

ALICEA SCHAEFFER, BS, RVT, VTS (Behavior), KPA CTP
Hillview Veterinary Clinic, Franklin, Indiana

BARBARA WATKINS, MA
Animal Keeper, Department of Animal Programs, Smithsonian's National Zoological Park, Washington, DC

MARGARET WHITTAKER, BS
Active Environments, Inc, Lompoc, California

Contents

> Behavior analysis is a data-driven science dedicated to understanding the mechanisms of behavior. Applied behavior analysis is a branch of this scientific field that systematically applies scientific principles to real-world problems in an effort to improve quality of life. The use of the behavioral technology provides a way to teach human and nonhuman animals more effectively and efficiently and offers those using this technology increased success in achieving behavioral goals.

> Animal training is an applied technology. Its foundation is rooted in the principles of behavior analysis. Understanding these principles of learning theory can be an important component of successful behavior modification; however, true behavior change is the result of practical application. Knowing the principles versus applying the technology are two very different skill sets. Animal trainers utilize a variety of specific tools, strategies and techniques to create a situation in which an animal will successfully learn to present a designated behavior. This article discusses the elements and process involved in the successful application of behavior change technology to create desired behaviors.

> Exotic animals are housed in a variety of settings, from pets at home, as display animals housed in wildlife centers and zoos, to those kept for interactive and outreach programs. The behavioral management program and medical care are major parts of an excellent animal care program. Because animals learn all the time, albeit through different mechanisms, animals are almost always "in training." Understanding animal learning when caring for and treating animals can greatly improve their welfare during experiences that are often related to involuntary procedures and where animals have little control over living conditions or procedures.

> Applied behavior analysis uses the understanding of behavioral mechanisms to manipulate the environment and effect behavior change. Functional assessments identify reinforcers maintaining problem behavior

using direct and indirect data collection strategies. After the function(s) of problem behavior have been confirmed or hypotheses have been made, interventions are designed and implemented. Behavior change strategies include antecedent interventions and training alternative behaviors that serve the same function as the problem behavior. Data are collected before, during, and after intervention, and all changes in treatment are based on these data.

The training of both domestic and exotic species for participation in medical behaviors is a helpful tool in the care and management of individual animals. The practice of training individual animals to help in their own health care is difficult to trace back to its origins. The use of these techniques on large exotic mammals became commonplace only as recently as the late 1990s and early 2000s. However, the practice seems to have been perfected and made popular with marine mammal species, starting in the 1970s. The development of better training techniques for a variety of medical behaviors is a foundational key worth examining and has been proven to be applicable across species.

In addition to being a large component of most zoological collections, reptile species are becoming more popular as family pets. Reptiles have the cognitive ability to be trained to facilitate daily husbandry and veterinary care. Desensitization and operant conditioning can alleviate some of the behavioral and physiological challenges of treating these species. A survey of reptile training programs at zoos in the United States and worldwide reveals that there are many successful training programs to facilitate veterinary care and minimize stress to the animal. Many of the techniques being used to train reptiles in zoological settings are transferable to the exotic pet clinician.

Nonhuman primates are excellent subjects for the enhancement of care and welfare through training. The application of positive reinforcement techniques to specific aspects of the management of captive nonhuman primates spans a wide range of species, social contexts, and housing situations (eg, laboratories, zoos, and sanctuaries). There is an increased interest from regulatory and accrediting agencies to insure improved conditions for captive nonhuman primates, apparent by the various standard guidelines, accreditation standards, and protocols available for the 3 primary types of nonhuman primate holding facilities.

Fishes and aquatic invertebrates are highly diverse groups of animals that are well adapted to their aquatic environments. For the past 200 years, researchers have been studying the learning potential of fishes and have shown them to be extensive. By using these animals' abilities to learn, caretakers can use operant conditioning with an emphasis on positive reinforcement to train behaviors aiding in dietary management, capture techniques, and medical procedures. Training fishes and aquatic invertebrates can help advance the care and well-being of these species in human care.

normal clinical appointment setting. However, this opportunity can still be used to introduce clients to the basics of training with positive reinforcement. These methods build a healthy relationship of trust between caregivers and their birds. Within the allotted appointment time, it is possible to teach clients how to train a simple behavior. This article outlines and demonstrates how training avian patients is successfully applied in a typical clinical practice.

Technicians, whose responsibilities are numerous, play a critical role in a veterinary practice. Clients need a trusted source for quality information on animal training and behavior that is based on science and noncoercive methods. The combination of addressing medical and behavioral needs of exotic animals allows a practice to provide added value for their clients. Technicians can play an important role in executing many aspects of a successful behavior program. From practical application in the examination room for hospitalized patients, to helping clients successfully train their animals at home, the end result is a cooperative patient and satisfied client.

VETERINARY CLINICS OF NORTH AMERICA: EXOTIC ANIMAL PRACTICE

THE CLINICS ARE NOW AVAILABLE ONLINE!
Access your subscription at:
www.theclinics.com

Preface

Exotic Animal Training and Learning

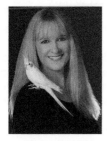

Barbara Heidenreich, BS(Zoology)
Guest Editor

Animal training and the learning theory behind it have become increasingly popular topics. Some textbooks and articles focus strictly on behavior analysis, some on behavioral natural history, and other more informal publications tend to focus on the practical application of training specific behaviors for specific species. Editing this publication provided an opportunity to combine all of these elements and more. Influencing animal behavior utilizes science, nature, and technique. Those who excel at creating behavioral change understand, practice, and draw on knowledge in all three areas.

Behavior analysis is a science that has been available to practitioners for more than 100 years. In the 1940s the Brelands took the information learned from the laboratory and started applying it in the real world with great success. Much of what animal trainers do in contemporary zoological settings today can be traced back to the Breland's operation and teachings.[1] Despite their pioneering efforts, a disconnect between academia and practical application still remains. Often we see behavior enthusiasts studying the science but lacking the hands-on experience with animals (or only applying it to human behavior). Understanding the definitions of the terms used in behavior analysis is very different from applying the principles to create behavior change in a wide variety of species.

On the other hand, there are also many self-proclaimed animal trainers that do not understand how they are influencing behavior. This type of trainer typically observes that their technique worked, but, without an understanding of learning theory, may not be using methods that contribute to high standards of animal welfare. This is what makes this publication a unique tool. Behavior analysis is the foundation, and all the authors speak from this same platform. However, each author was also chosen to help bridge the gap between scientific knowledge and how to use it to get desired behavior while at the same time attending to high animal welfare standards.

Vet Clin Exot Anim 15 (2012) xi–xii
http://dx.doi.org/10.1016/j.cvex.2012.06.013 **vetexotic.theclinics.com**

While it can be argued that all organisms are governed by the "laws" of behavior and therefore training is the same across species, without a doubt trainers employ specific techniques, use different tools, and change their approach with different taxonomic groups. The principles of behavior analysis used to address a common problem may be the same, but the technique will be different. What a reptile finds reinforcing may be vastly different from a rabbit or a bird. Working with some species may require a trainer to accommodate social dynamics in order to have a successful training session. Other species may be more likely to respond to training when a place to hide is included in the training area. Experienced animal trainers know this attention to subtle detail is important to successfully achieve behavior goals.

Training is also a mechanical skill. Being prepared to deliver reinforcers in direct conjunction with behavior, knowing when to raise or relax criteria, and having excellent observational skills are all elements of training that are learned by practice. Practitioners seeking to improve their technique will find information in this publication to help them fine tune their skills.

Real behavior change is the result of practical application. This publication is designed to help those with an interest in utilizing the science of behavior analysis and the experience of those who practice its application everyday with animals in real-life conditions to help improve the welfare of the animals in their care. Animal training provides undeniable benefits when it comes to health care for the animals we steward. This publication includes many examples of how animal training has been used to facilitate health care in species ranging from fish, birds, reptiles, primates, rabbits, guinea pigs, and more. It is my hope that veterinary professionals will be inspired by the examples and teachings within this publication and become pioneers willing to explore the potential of science-based training technology and how it applies to medical care. The merging of animal training and medical care is in the early stages of development. There is an exciting future ahead as animal care professionals continue to explore how training can be incorporated into veterinary medicine.

Barbara Heidenreich, BS(Zoology)
Good Bird, Inc.
PO Box 150604
Austin, TX 78715, USA

E-mail address:
info@goodbirdinc.com

REFERENCE

1. Bailey R, Gillaspy J. Operant psychology goes to the fair. Marian and Keller Breland in the popular press, 1947-1966. Behav Analyst 2005;28:143–59.

Behavior Analysis
The Science of Training

Parvene Farhoody, MA

KEYWORDS

- Behavior analysis • Applied behavior analysis • Operant conditioning
- Three-term contingency • Behavioral technology • Science of behavior

KEY POINTS

- Behavior analysis is the science of behavior change.
- A systematic approach to teaching behavior and changing behavior improves effectiveness and efficiency.
- Operational definitions and quantifiable measurement of behavior are defining features of applied behavior analysis.
- Behavior analysts work with human and nonhuman species to improve quality of life.

INTRODUCTION

Behavior analysis is the science of behavior change. B.F. Skinner defined this distinct branch of natural science in the 1930s with his introduction of the 3-term contingency. Behavior analysts are interested in measuring observable behavior to discover functional relationships between the environment and behavior. Behavior analysis is divided into 2 branches: the experimental analysis of behavior (EAB) and applied behavior analysis (ABA). EAB focuses on behavior as a phenomenon, and work is generally conducted in laboratory settings, whereas ABA generally uses empirical data collected in real-world settings to systematically apply behavioral principles to effect behavior change. A systematic approach to behavior change is a defining feature of behavior analysis and distinguishes it from other science-based approaches to behavior. Another defining feature of behavior analysis is the use of operational definitions of behavior. A behavior that is operationally defined has been described in such clear observational terms that anyone can recognize when the behavior is happening or not happening. Operational definitions make it possible to measure behavior objectively and accurately. Operational definitions also eliminate constructs as descriptions

The author has nothing to disclose.
Department of Psychology, Queens College, Graduate Center of the City University of New York, 65-30 Kissena Boulevard Flushing, NY 11367, USA
E-mail addresses: parvene@behaviormatters.com; pfarhoody@gc.cuny.edu

Vet Clin Exot Anim 15 (2012) 361–369
http://dx.doi.org/10.1016/j.cvex.2012.06.001
1094-9194/12/$ – see front matter © 2012 Elsevier Inc. All rights reserved.

of behavior. These labels do not provide the necessary information for analyzing behavior with precision. ABA practitioners hold a master's or doctoral degree in behavior analysis or have completed a formal education in a program approved by the Behavior Analyst Certification Board (BACB).

In the last chapter of *The Behavior of Organisms,* B.F. Skinner states, "Operant behavior with its unique relation to the environment presents a separate important field of investigation."[1(p438)] This began a distinct branch of psychology called the EAB. In this field of psychology, behavior is viewed as a natural science, comparable to mathematics and physics. As with other natural sciences, the emphasis is on empirical findings. However, what most distinguishes behavior analysis from other branches of psychology is its emphasis on analysis of data collected through the direct observation of measurable behavior.[2,3] It is important to note that behavior analysts do not deny the existence of mental processes (emotions, memories, and so forth) as influences on behavior. In fact, unlike behavior scientists before him, such as Ernst Mach and J. B. Watson, Skinner acknowledged mental process. "When we say that behavior is a function of the environment, the term 'environment' presumably means any event in the universe capable of affecting the organism. But part of the universe is enclosed within the organism's own skin."[4(p257)] However, Skinner's work followed a long history of the use of introspection to study mental processes, and in order to remove his work from this subjectivity, he committed himself to study only behavior that could be directly measured. To the behavior analyst, any observable behavior is of interest; this includes all overt or outwardly observable behavior as well as biological behavior that can be directly measured, such as breathing rate, heart rate, or cortisol levels.

THE THREE-TERM CONTINGENCY

Skinner's great contribution was the 3-term contingency.[1,5] As with any natural phenomenon, Skinner did not discover that there was a relationship between environmental events and behavior in the sense that he created it; he discovered this behavioral phenomenon just as Newton discovered gravity. Skinner recognized that certain behavioral phenomena obeyed laws, and by understanding those laws, he was able to make predictions about outcomes. The 3-term contingency can be viewed as the formula used to make predictions about behavior. Newton made predictions about how the planets moved, and Skinner made predictions about how behavior occurred. Each scientist based his predictions on existing physical phenomena. Behavior is lawful, and the universal principles are based on the functional relationships that exist between what happens immediately before and immediately after a behavior. The principles are universal in the sense that they apply across species. This does not mean that all animals are the same; it simply means that all animals respond to behavioral principles in a similar manner. The gravitational forces that keep humans from flying off the planet are the same gravitational forces that keep rats, horses, and dogs from flying off the planet. Behavior is a cross-species phenomenon.

The 3-term contingency, in symbolic form, is expressed as:

$$S^D : R_1 \rightarrow S^R$$

The presentation of a discriminative stimulus (S^D; this is colloquially referred to as a cue) sets the occasion for a response (R_1) that leads to the availability of a consequence (S^R).[1] A simpler way to express this equation is A:B $\rightarrow$ C, where A stands for Antecedent, B for Behavior, and C for Consequence. This is sometimes referred to as the ABCs of behavior analysis.[2] The contingent relationship among these 3 events (antecedent, behavior, and consequence) is the 3-term contingency. This relationship is said to be functional because it can be predicted that the consequence is always contingent on the behavior being performed and that the behavior does not occur unless preceded by the antecedent. In other words, the manipulation of one event can reliably predict a change in another event. In the simplest terms: if this happens, then that happens. In behavior analysis, the smallest unit of behavior is the 3-term contingency.[6]

OPERANT VERSUS CLASSIC CONDITIONING

Once Skinner's operant conditioning 3-term contingency defined the basic unit of learning, it became possible to examine the operant learning process with the same scientific rigor that had previously been applied to examining classic conditioning.[7,8] Skinner defined the difference between Pavlovian or classic conditioning and operant conditioning: Pavlovian conditioning occurs when an association is made between a stimulus and a response. This usually occurs when a neutral stimulus is presented immediately before an unconditioned stimulus. The relationship between the antecedent and the response is a 2-term contingency represented as $S \rightarrow R$. The presentation of the stimulus *causes* the behavior to occur. In Pavlov's classic experiments, a bell rings and the dog salivates; the antecedent (the bell) *causes* the response (salivation).[9] The dog has no control over his response; it is elicited by the sound of the bell. In operant conditioning, it is the *consequence* that most influences the response. The antecedent merely sets the occasion for a response to occur. The consequence will occur only if the animal gives the appropriate response. In operant conditioning, the behavior of the animal determines whether or not the consequence occurs; the animal operates on its environment. For example, a target stick is presented, the rabbit places its nose on the target stick, and food is delivered. The rabbit responds to the antecedent and the consequence is presented contingent on that response. The presentation of the target stick did not *cause* the rabbit to place its nose on it. The rabbit *chooses* to put its nose on the target stick because of what it has learned about the relationship between placing its nose on the target stick and a consequence. It is the consequence that most influences the response. In the operant conditioning paradigm, *behavior is a function of its consequences.* Skinner's 3-term contingency was the $E = mc^2$ of behavior science.

THE FOUR-TERM CONTINGENCY

In recent years, a 4-term contingency has been proposed that considers the motivational state of the organism as part of the behavioral equation. Motivating operations are unconditioned or conditioned antecedent stimuli that increase or decrease the value of a reinforcer or any behavior that has led to that reinforcer in the past. A very simplistic example would be the following: thirst is a motivating operation that increases the value of water as a reinforcer and also increases the behavior of drinking out of a water fountain, because that behavior has led to access to water in the past. This fourth variable is placed before the ABC and provides information about the *probability* that a behavior will occur within the 3-term contingency. For those ABA practitioners working with nonhuman species, the potential of this extended analysis offers exciting possibilities for predicting and controlling behavioral outcomes. It is mentioned here as a subject worthy of examination. For more information on the 4-term contingency and the complex relationship between motivating operations and behavior, see Michael[10] and Keller and Schoenfeld.[11]

QUANTIFYING BEHAVIOR

Behavior can be examined only when the behavior, antecedent, and consequence are clearly defined. In a sense, the question, "My dog jumps on me; what do I do?" does not provide the information necessary to answer the question. Along the same lines, a dog that perceives a biscuit in the environment and subsequently goes through an entire repertoire of behaviors, such as sit, down, roll over, spin, bark, and so forth, is exhibiting an indiscriminate response repertoire unrelated to the supposed cues (the spoken words *sit*, *down*, *spin*, etc). This is quite different from behavior that is in response to specific discriminative stimuli (ie, the behavior is "on cue"). In other words, the sit behavior may occur when the biscuit is present, but the behaviors down and spin may also occur. The indiscriminate behavior exhibited by the dog also indicates that the supposed cues for sit, down, and so forth are unlikely to be functionally related to the occurrence of the behavior, meaning the dog has not discriminated that the sound "sit" is the greatest predictor of reinforcement. It fact, given the behavior exhibited, it is most likely that the dog has discriminated that the presence of the biscuit is the best predictor of reinforcement, which is why the frequency of those behaviors increased as soon as the dog perceived the presence of the biscuit. To the behavior analyst, these differences are not subtle. Observable, measurable dimensions define a behavior; therefore, the accuracy of the response in terms of salience of a discriminative stimulus, frequency of response, latency of response, stimulus generalization, and response generalization are just a few of the behavioral parameters that require attention when planning and implementing teaching protocols.

This quantitative specificity is an essential feature of behavior analysis and one that distinguishes a behavior analysis approach from that of other teaching paradigms. Behavior analysis is not a philosophy or method of training; it is the systematic application of behavioral principles to effect behavior change. At its core, behavior analysis is the "science of behavior change."[12(p4)] A more formal definition might be "a field of inquiry devoted to investigation factors that influence behavior in a systematic way— the science of behavior."[3(p3)] A definition of *applied* behavior analysis is "the science in which tactics derived from the principles of behavior are applied systematically to improve socially significant behavior and experimentation is used to identify the variables responsible for behavior change."[2(p20)]

SKINNER AND DARWIN

At the time of Skinner's work, Darwin's theory of evolution had taken hold in the scientific community, and the idea that "function" played a large part in evolution greatly influenced Skinner. Darwinian evolution proposed that when an organism's physical attributes allowed it to function successfully within a given environment and survive, the organism would live on to reproduce and pass on the functional features to its offspring.[13] Skinner translated this process of natural selection to learning and viewed the principles governing the operant conditioning process as selection by consequences. Successful behaviors that lead to desired consequences are repeated and maintained within a behavioral repertoire, and those that do not lead to desired consequences become extinct.[1,14]

THE PROGRESSION OF BEHAVIOR ANALYSIS

From the late 1930s on, behavior analysts continued their study of the functional relationships between environmental events and behavior. In 1949, P.R. Fuller applied the principles of operant conditioning to a human subject. A man in a vegetative state was taught to raise his arm using warm milk as a reinforcer.[15] Fuller published an article discussing his findings in the *American Journal of Psychology* and so began a new direction for behavior analysis: the application of behavioral principles to improve the lives of human beings. The translation of behavioral principles into applied settings with the goal of improving human lives became known as the field of applied behavior analysis, which formally began in 1959 with the publication of "The Psychiatric Nurse as a Behavioral Engineer."[16] The article discussed how to use behavioral principles to improve the lives of residents in a psychiatric institution. From the 1950s through the 1980s, the field of behavior analysis expanded exponentially in the direction of applying behavioral principles discovered in the laboratory to human behavior. During that time, ABA concentrated mostly in the areas of developmental disabilities and education.

Today, there are 2 main branches of behavior analysis: the EAB and ABA.

- Experimental behavior analysts study behavior as a phenomenon. In the tradition of Skinner, these behavior analysts generally work in laboratory settings conducting controlled experiments with human and nonhuman participants. This work continues to advance the science, and expand our understanding of how behavior works, by building on the existing body of knowledge gained through scientific experimentation over the past 120 years. The research from this branch of behavioral science is published in the field's professional journal, *The Journal of the Experimental Analysis of Behavior*.
- ABA practitioners generally apply the science of behavior in real-life settings. Because the application of science is considered technology, ABA practitioners are said to use behavioral technology to effect behavior change. The vast majority of the recipients of the services of ABA practitioners continues to be those who are developmentally disabled, such as those with autism, psychiatric disorders, or cognitive impairment (such as brain injury), or those in need of specialized assistance in learning. The work of ABA practitioners requires direct teaching of the person whose behavior is being changed as well as working with the person's caregivers regarding how to implement and maintain the teaching protocols provided by the practitioner. The peer-reviewed findings of the behavioral technology conducted in applied settings are found in *The Journal of Applied Behavior Analysis*.

BEHAVIOR ANALYSIS VERSUS OTHER SCIENTIFIC APPROACHES

A definition of *science* is a systematic approach to the understanding of natural phenomenon as evidenced by description, prediction, and control, that relies on determinism as it fundamental assumption, empiricism as its prime directive, experimentation as its basic strategy, replication as its necessary requirement for believability, parsimony as its conservative value and philosophical doubt as its guiding conscience.[2]

The term "science-based training" has become a catch-all phrase in animal training, so it is important to define what is meant by behavior analysis or behavioral technology. An applied behavior analyst measures observable behavior to discover functional relationships between the environment and behavior, and he or she then systematically applies behavioral principles to change behavior. Of course, anyone who is changing any behavior is theoretically using behavioral principles, because behavior can only change according to learning principles. However, the difference lies in the extent to which the behavioral technician is aware of the mechanisms being used. Behavior analysis is a data-driven science and uses direct measurement to assess behavior change.[17] Only through objective measurement and analysis can teaching become a technology that can be replicated and improved through the scientific process of peer review. This is true when building a new behavior or solving a behavior problem. As with a medical treatment, decisions about interventions are based on empirical information. Measurements are taken at baseline, and treatment plans are designed and implemented according to quantitative data. After any intervention, behavioral outcomes are measured and compared with baseline in order to assess the intervention's success or failure. If improvements in the form of increases, decreases, or maintenance of the desired behaviors are not observed, procedures are altered accordingly. For an interesting discussion of the philosophy and science of behavior analysis as a distinct field of study, see Chiesa.[18]

As with all good science, behavior analysis begins with objectivity. This starts with the definition of behavior. As mentioned previously, behavior analysis looks at overt behavior; behaviors targeted for change are given an operational definition. This requires describing a behavior's topography in great detail. An operationally defined behavior is one that has been described in such clear observational terms that anyone can recognize when the behavior is happening or not happening. Operational definitions of behavior make it possible to measure behavior objectively and accurately.[3] Behavior analysts will always describe behavior only in terms of what they can see, measure, and verify. One can often differentiate behavior analysts from any other sort of behaviorist or trainer by the way they describe behavior.

HYPOTHETICAL CONSTRUCTS AND EXPLANATORY FICTIONS

When behavior is not described objectively or cannot be easily explained, it is common to turn to hypothetical constructs or explanatory fictions. Constructs are labels or stories about a behavior that do not describe behavior. They are fictitious variables that do not lead to an understanding of the actual variables responsible for the development of the behavior or to an understanding of the environmental events that are maintaining the behavior.[2] Constructs include words such as *stubborn*, *lazy*, *spoiled*, *stupid*, *dominant*, *spiteful*, or *intelligent*, *friendly*, *sweet*, and *likes to please*. None of these constructions describes a behavior. Humans often use hypothetical constructs to rationalize behavior that has not been clearly or operationally defined. Constructs can lead to the perception of unexplained behavior as mysterious, unpredictable, or irrational. Explanatory fictions are circular, unverifiable arguments, such as: Why does the rat press the lever? Because he is hungry. How do you know the rat is hungry? Because he presses the lever.

Behavior analysis avoids hypothetical constructs and explanatory fictions for several reasons:

1. *There is a loss of scientific objectivity.* Construct and explanatory fictions cannot be measured. If a change in behavior cannot be objectively measured before any treatment is given, there are no empirical data to assess the effects of the treatment, and therefore assessment of treatment becomes arbitrary and subjective.
2. *Any number of behaviors could fit into one construction.* A parrot described as "hormonal" could exhibit a number of behaviors that make the human describe her this way. The parrot could be engaging in nesting behavior, biting a nonpreferred family member, or screaming. A precise definition is critical for precision in training and solving problems. In behavior analysis, the goal is to change behavior efficiently and effectively in the direction desired, as a result of the controlled

manipulation of measurable variables, not to rely on a hit-or-miss process that eventually arrives at some change in behavior.

3. *The use of constructs and explanatory fictions validates often emotionally charged interpretations of behavior.* This is very important when dealing with human caregivers. When stories are given as the reason for behavior, the caregiver continues to concentrate on unprovable explanations, which can lead to complacency. Constructs tend to lead to the belief that a training or behavior problem somehow lies within the animal rather than being caused by environmental factors that can be changed through the systematic application of learning principles.

4. *In the science of behavior analysis, behavior is viewed as deterministic, as a product of cause-and-effect relationships.* This is perhaps the most important reason that explanatory fictions and constructs are not in the behavior analyst's vernacular. Functional relationships exist between behavior and the environment. Behavior is maintained because it serves a function for the animal; it has an effect. The first job of the behavior analyst is to determine the function of a behavior. This allows for further analysis and accuracy in changing behavior. *(See the article by Farhoody elsewhere in this issue titled, A Framework for Solving Behavior Problems.)*

BEHAVIOR 101

The difficulty with viewing behavior as a science that can be approached systematically is that behavior occurs, changes, and is manipulated all the time, without any particular awareness on the part of the creature whose behavior changes. Every moment of every day is filled with innumerable behavior and behavior changes. A trip to the grocery store, a dog eliminates outdoors, a student graduates from high school, a boss threatens to fire a late employee: all of these are examples of behavior in constant motion. How each of these large and small behavior changes occurred, as the result of the relationship between individual behaviors and the environment, is not regularly analyzed or identified, yet the functional relationships that were responsible can be analyzed and determined. The fact that the behavior was acquired or changed is not the only important information; the behavior analyst is interested in the processes by which the behavior was acquired, the length of time it took to learn the behavior, the willingness of the participant to engage in the behavior, the behavior's resistance to change or extinction, the manner in which the behavior will be maintained, and the method by which to teach others to maintain the behavior, to name but a few.[2,19–21]

The basic learning principles, sometimes called the 4 quadrants, are the tip of the behavior science iceberg. Most people are familiar with these basic learning principles: positive and negative reinforcement and positive and negative punishment. These basic principles are covered in every Psychology 101 course, behavior textbook, and most any animal training–type class. Although the basic principles are a very good place to start, knowing what these principles are is only the beginning. Knowing that deoxygenated blood enters the right atrium of the heart and flows into the right ventricle is a good place to start, but it does not make you a cardiologist. The 4 quadrants is an introduction to behavior science. Understanding the mechanisms by which these behavioral principles effect change is fundamental to a systematic approach to behavior change. On top of all this, a good behavior analyst must have the mechanical skill necessary to apply those behavioral principles under real-world conditions, skills that can come only from hands-on application. Behavior analysis has moved far beyond the Skinner box in the last 60 years. Assessment of behavior problems and treatment strategies are now used as part of a continually expanding behavioral technology. The speed and accuracy with which typically developing subjects can learn even complex behavior have allowed for development of human and animal potential. Behavioral technology continues to develop as derived behavioral principles, concepts, and procedures are refined. Behavioral economics, behavioral momentum, behavioral contrast, matching law, law of diminishing returns, timing effects, fluency, token economies, and many other empirically derived and tested theories are now broadening our understanding of how behavior is acquired, changed, and maintained and how we can use these behavioral principles to improve teaching on every level. This is reflected in the expansion of ABA over the last 30 years into areas such as organizational behavior management, self-control, addiction, crime prevention and rehabilitation, delinquency and forensic behavior analysis, direct instruction, behavioral medicine, behavioral coaching and counseling, gambling, parenting, speech pathology, pediatric feeding disorders, health, sports, fitness, and applied animal behavior, among many others. Today, a few ABA practitioners are turning their attention to animals or, more precisely, back to animals, because nonhuman animals were the behavioral models from which the analysis of behavior began. For a comprehensive examination of the history of applied animal behavior, see Bailey and Gillaspy.[22]

STANDARD PRACTICES

Today, applied behavior analysts are held to standards established by the BACB. These include educational and standard practices, as well as ethical and humane guidelines. Master's and doctoral degrees can be attained in behavior analysis working with any species. Since 1998, those working with humans and meeting all the requirements set forth by the BACB can earn the designation board-certified behavior analyst. Requirements include a minimum of a master's degree in behavior analysis or other natural science; completing 1500 hours of applied work, 75 hours of which must be under the supervision of a board-certified behavior analyst; and then taking a standardized examination. The understanding that it is necessary to complete a formal education in the field of behavior and to have supervised practice in application to be considered a specialist qualified to work with humans with special needs is not surprising. However, the same standards are still relatively unexpected when working with nonhuman species. Perhaps because of this, only those who work with humans may take the board certification exam at this time. Those who work exclusively with nonhuman species may not take the exam even if they have met all other requirements. Special interest groups within the field of ABA, such as those within the Association for Behavior Analysis International, are diligently working to demonstrate that the humane standards and ethical and professional guidelines applied to humans can and should apply to work with nonhuman species. Once accomplished, this will be another great step forward in advancing the field of behavior analysis to improve the lives of humans whose work revolves around improving the lives of the nonhuman species in their care.

SUMMARY

This brief introduction was intended to provide a basic overview of the branch of science called behavior analysis. A systematic approach to changing behavior may at first glance seem needlessly tedious. After all, behavior can be changed using many approaches. However, the time and dedication put into learning to use behavioral technology bring the rewards of speed and accuracy in training and reduced stress to both teacher and student as a result. Much like learning to use a computer, it may be hard at first, but soon it is hard to know how you ever lived without it when it comes to the efficiency with which things can get done The companion article else-where in this issue continues the discussion of behavior analysis with the examination of the behavior-analytic approach to changing behavior.

REFERENCES

1. Skinner BF. The behavior of organisms. New York: Appleton-Century-Crofts; 1938.
2. Cooper JO, Heron TE, Heward WL. Applied behavior analysis. 2nd edition. Upper Saddle River (NJ): Pearson Education; 2007.
3. Sulzer-Azaroff B, Mayer GR. Behavior analysis for lasting change. Orlando (FL): Harcourt Brace College Publishers; 1991.
4. Skinner BF. Science and human behavior. New York: MacMillan; 1953.
5. Ferster CB, Skinner BF. Schedules of reinforcement. Acton (MA): Copley Publishing Group; 1957.
6. Thompson T, Lubinski D. Units of analysis and kinetic structure of behavioral repertoires. J Exp Anal Behav 1986;469:219–42.
7. Anrep GV. The irradiation of conditioned reflexes. Proc R Soc Lond Biol Sci 1923; 94:404–26.
8. Bass MJ, Hull C. The irradiation of a tactile conditioned reflex in man. J Comp Psychol 1934;17:47–65.
9. Pavlov IP. Conditioned reflexes. Anrep GP, trans. London: Oxford University Press; 1927.
10. Michael J. Distinguishing between discriminative and motivational functions of stimuli. J Exp Anal Behav 1982;37:149–55.
11. Keller FS, Schoenfeld WN. Principles of psychology: a systematic text in the science of behavior. Century psychology series. East Norwalk (CT): Appleton-Century-Crofts; 1950. p. 262–325.
12. Chance P. First course in applied behavior analysis. Pacific Grove (CA): Brooks/ Cole; 1998.
13. Darwin C. On the origin of species. 6th edition. London: John Murray and Co; 1872.
14. Skinner BF. Selection by consequences. Science 1981;213:501–4.
15. Fuller PR. Operant conditioning of a vegetative organism. Am J Psychol 1949;62: 587–90.
16. Ayllon T, Azrin NH. The psychiatric nurse as a behavioral engineer. J Exp Anal Behav 1959;2:323–34.
17. Cooper JO. Measuring behavior. 2nd edition. Columbus (OH): Charles E. Merrill Publishing; 1981.
18. Chiesa M. Radical behaviorism: the philosophy and the science. Sarasota (FL): Authors Cooperative; 1994.
19. Terrace HS. Discrimination learning with and without errors. J Exp Anal Behav 1963;6:1–27.
20. Lindsley OR. Precision teaching: discoveries and effects. J Appl Behav Anal 1992;25:51–7.
21. Mazur JE. Learning and behavior. 6th edition. Upper Saddle River (NJ): Pearson; 2006.
22. Bailey RE, Gillaspy JA Jr. Operant psychology goes to the fair: Marian and Keller Breland in the popular press, 1947-1966. Behav Anal 2005;28:143–59.

An Introduction to the Application of Science-Based Training Technology

Barbara Heidenreich, BS(Zoology)

KEYWORDS

- Animal training • Positive reinforcement • Behavior change technology
- Shaping with approximations • Capturing behavior • Reinforcers

KEY POINTS

- Empowerment of the animal to choose to be a voluntary participant is a critical component in training animals to cooperate in their own medical care.
- Conscientious trainers focus on using positive reinforcement.
- Effective animal trainers aim for creating an environment in which the animal will likely be receptive to a training session.
- To facilitate clear communication and faster training, it is also important to train one behavior at a time.
- It is very important to avoid creating fear responses in successful animal training for medical behaviors.

 Videos of training of a guinea hog, elephant, giraffe, parrots, and guinea pig accompanies this article http://www.vetexotic.theclinics.com/.

POSITIVE REINFORCEMENT TRAINING

Training is essentially a form of communication. It has structure and mechanics and is procedural in nature. When a systematic approach is applied to teaching, the end result is clear communication from trainer to animal. It makes it more likely an animal will understand what actions earn desired consequences.

Although animal behavior can be modified using many of the principles of behavior analysis, contemporary animal trainers focus on the use of the least intrusive, most positive methods. This means aversives are not considered an appropriate tool for influencing animal behavior. While they are effective, research has demonstrated that coercion and the use of aversives have fallout; this can include the presentation

The author has nothing to disclose.
Good Bird Inc, PO Box 150604, Austin, TX 78715, USA
E-mail address: Barb@GoodBirdInc.com

Vet Clin Exot Anim 15 (2012) 371–385
http://dx.doi.org/10.1016/j.cvex.2012.06.006
1094-9194/12/$ – see front matter © 2012 Published by Elsevier Inc.

of escape, avoidance, and aggressive behaviors.[1] This empowerment of the animal to choose to be a voluntary participant is a critical component in training animals to cooperate in their own medical care.

To effectively train new behaviors and maintain a relationship based on trust with an animal, conscientious trainers focus on using positive reinforcement. Reinforcement is the procedure of providing consequences for a behavior that increases or maintains the frequency of that behavior.[2] Positive reinforcement indicates something is added to the environment to increase the designated behavior. In animal training, positive reinforcers tend to be things the animal seeks to acquire or values. This can include items such as preferred food, access to enrichment items, tactile, companionship, and, in some cases, verbal responses from caregivers.

Although animal training is derived from behavior analysis, the terminology typically used can often be colloquial. **Table 1** describes a few terms commonly used in practical application and their scientific equivalent.

CREATING THE DESIRED BEHAVIOR

The first step in training a desired behavior is creating an action to reinforce. This requires having a clear picture of what the presentation of the desired behavior will look like once trained. In most situations, the animal will not have history of presenting the desired action and getting reinforced. Therefore, trainers have to create a step or approximation toward that goal behavior that can be reinforced. For example, to train a parrot to allow nail trimming without restraint, a first approximation may be for the bird to lift its foot. A parrot that has experience stepping onto hands for positive reinforcement may lift a foot when a hand is presented close to its feet. Rather than waiting for the bird to step up, the trainer can reinforce the parrot the exact moment the foot is lifted from the perch. This creates an opportunity for the desired first approximation to be reinforced.

There are numerous ways to create a desired action that do not involve coercion. A common tool in animal training is a target. The action of orienting a body part toward a target is called *targeting*.[3(p15)] Once an animal has learned to target, it is possible to use the target to direct the animal where to go or where to place a body part. This allows the trainer to give the animal information and create action that can be reinforced without having to handle or manipulate the animal. For example, another way to train a parrot to lift its foot for nail trimming is to train it to touch a target with its foot. To train a lion to allow intramuscular injections, the target may be used to train the lion to press its hip against the mesh of the enclosure to allow easy access for the procedure. A target can also be used to direct an animal to walk into a crate or chute. In this example, the animal may be trained to orient its nose or beak toward the target.

Table 1	
Animal training terminology and the equivalent behavior analysis terminology	
Animal Training Terminology	**Behavior Analysis Terminology**
Cue	Discriminative stimulus
Bridge or event marker	Conditioned reinforcer
Time out	Negative punishment
Motivation, hunger	Motivating operations
On cue	Under stimulus control
Behavior is solid	Behavior is fluent

Animals quickly learn to move in the direction of the target to earn reinforcers. Targeting can have many applications in creating an action that can be reinforced (**Fig. 1**, Videos 1 and 2 (online at www.vetexotic.theclinics.com)).

Action can also be created by showing reinforcers. For example, a guinea pig may climb up onto a scale in response to the smell or sight of a carrot resting on top. If this action is reinforced by the opportunity to eat the carrot, the animal can learn to repeat the behavior in the future whenever a scale is present. Over time, the presence of the scale will indicate the opportunity exists to earn access to a carrot. The carrot will no longer need to be seen or smelled for the animal to present the behavior. Once the animal climbs onto the scale, the carrot can be delivered.

Fading out showing the reinforcer helps prevent the animal from becoming dependent on seeing or smelling the reinforcer before presenting the behavior. This can be especially important if a situation requires the animal does not eat, for example, to avoid aspiration when anesthetized. A strong reinforcement history for this behavior will help keep it resistant to extinction when food reinforcers must be withheld on rare occasions for procedures. Other strategies trainers use to avoid aspiration are to use nonfood reinforcers or use frozen liquid reinforcers that can be licked to reduce the quantities consumed yet still reinforce the behavior (such as goat's milk or blood for exotic cats).

SHAPING WITH APPROXIMATIONS

Once an action or approximation toward the desired behavior is created and reinforced, the trainer focuses on building more behavior using targets, showing reinforcers or careful observation of the animal's action. If the animal makes any action that builds upon the previous action, the trainer reinforces that action. Each approximation that is successfully reinforced brings the animal closer to presenting the desired final behavior.

The trainer's objective is to make it as easy as possible for the animal to present the next step or approximation. If the animal fails to move to the next approximation after 2 to 3 attempts, it is the trainer's responsibility to relax the criteria so that the animal can successfully earn a reinforcer. This is often referred to as asking for a smaller approximation or less behavior.

Identifying smaller approximations can be difficult for inexperienced trainers. People tend to be focused on obtaining the goal behavior as opposed to making the approximations easily mastered by the animal. Pushing for too much behavior can lead to an animal

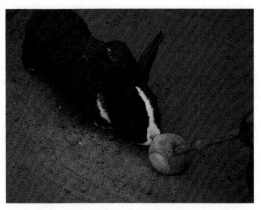

Fig. 1. A rabbit targets to a tennis ball. This allows the trainer to direct the animal where to go without the use of coercion.

losing interest in the training session as it is unable to earn the reinforcer. It can also lead to aggressive behavior, especially when the animal is highly motivated for the reinforcers, which are not forthcoming because the criterion is too high.

Conversely, if an animal has presented an approximation successfully repeatedly, it is important to move onto the next approximation. Repeating the same approximation more than 3 times can lead to a history of reinforcement for that approximation. This increases the likelihood the animal will continue to repeat that same approximation as opposed to offering additional behavior in order to earn a reinforcer.

Obtaining behaviors may require progressing through a variety of approximations. These steps should be approached systematically. When 1 step is mastered, the next step is attempted. Each approximation adds new criteria for the animal to learn or allow.

Because training technology is a form of communication attempting to add more than 1 criterion at a time can be detrimental to the process. For example, if a parrot is being trained to lift its foot, the final behavior may have the criterion that the foot is held at a certain height for 30 seconds. Rather than trying to reinforce for increased height and increased duration during a session, focus is on training for 1 criterion, such as the desired height. Shaping for duration is added after height has been trained to fluency.

BRIDGING STIMULUS

The reinforcer is the tool that communicates to the animal it has presented behavior desired by the trainer. It is important that delivery of the reinforcer is paired in direct conjunction with the presentation of the desired action.[3(p69)] This clear communication is dependent on excellent observational skills and timing on the part of the trainer. The moment the desired action is observed is the moment a reinforcer should be delivered for most effective communication.

Trainers should be prepared to deliver reinforcers immediately. This means having reinforcers readily available in a pocket, pouch, hand, or other readily accessible container. Some trainers discreetly load reinforcers into their fingertips while the animal is working so they are ready to reinforce. Others will use another trainer just to reinforce the animal if necessary. Timing of the delivery of the reinforcer is critical for clear communication from trainer to animal.

Some behaviors require trainers to work at a distance from the animal. In these situations it is not possible to deliver the reinforcer in direction conjunction with the presentation of the behavior. Under such circumstances a trainer will use a bridging stimulus (bridge) or event marker. The bridge is a sound or signal the animal has learned marks the desired action and indicates reinforcers will be delivered or available momentarily.[3(p70)] Research has shown that the bridge only affords the trainer a limited extra amount of time to deliver the reinforcer. Waiting too long to deliver the reinforcer can cause presentation of undesired behavior and/or a failure in communication.[4]

Although the bridge does precede the delivery of the reinforcer, it should be presented when the trainer observes the action desired. Trainers are advised to practice the timing of the presentation of the bridge to ensure it occurs at the exact moment the behavior is observed. It is a common practice for novice trainers to present the bridge just before delivering reinforcers as opposed to marking behavior observed.

Bridges are also useful when action is being presented quickly. A skilled observer can mark the desired action in the midst of a stream of behaviors being presented. If the desired action is marked consistently and reinforced, the animal can learn which of the many behaviors presented is being bridged and earned the reinforcers.

Once understood by the animal, bridges tend to halt behavior and redirect attention toward obtaining the reinforcer. Many animals will show body language indicative of anticipating the reinforcer when the event marker is presented. This is another reason excellent observation skills and good timing are important. Animals also tend to notice any sound or action that may indicate a reinforcer is about to be delivered. For this reason, many trainers are quiet and still until the moment the bridge is presented. Reaching into a pocket for a food reinforcer before giving an event marker can be enough to bridge a behavior.

Commonly used bridges are clickers, whistles, and specific words, such as "good," "yes," or "OK." Other signals such as a light or touch can also acts as event markers. The bridge signal is learned by the animal during the training process. The experience of presenting action, receiving the bridge followed by a reinforcer gives the bridge significance to the animal.

Bridges are a tool to help mark behavior when it is difficult to deliver reinforcers promptly. They are not required under all training circumstances. Once a behavior is trained to fluency, bridges are no longer necessary to maintain the behavior. They can be faded out. However, reinforcers should not be faded out as they are critical to maintaining behaviors.

CUES

Cues are sounds or signals that indicate the opportunity exists to present an action and earn reinforcers. Cues acquire their value by being paired with the action followed by the reinforcer. Sounds and signals are meaningless as cues without this pairing.

Once a behavior or action has been created and reinforced, an animal will start to present the behavior without being prompted by targets or other tools in order to earn desired reinforcers. This is commonly referred to as offering the behavior. When an animal begins to offer behavior, the trainer can usually anticipate the next presentation of the action. In those moments that precede the presentation of the behavior a trainer can present the cue. If the animal presents the behavior within a few seconds of the presentation of the cue, the trainer reinforces the behavior. This process is repeated to build history of reinforcement for presenting the behavior after the cue. At this point in the process, the trainer no longer reinforces the animal for offering the behavior. When the animal consistently presents the behavior after the presentation of the cue and can discriminate between different cued behaviors, the behavior is considered to be on cue or under stimulus control.[3(p74)]

Cues can be any sound or signal the trainer chooses. While many choose to use words that describe the behavior, such as "step up," "station," or "scale," it is important to note that any word or signal could be used. The word gains meaning via the reinforcement process.

Sounds or signals can also be used to give information to an animal that a procedure is about to happen. Some medical procedures involve pain or tactile to body parts animals cannot see. For example, drawing blood from the back of an elephant's ear may cause pain. The elephant also cannot see the needle when it is inserted into the vein. An elephant can quickly learn to associate the instruments and circumstances involved with blood draws with anticipation of pain. This can increase anxiety as the elephant waits for needle insertion. This can lead to the animal breaking position or breakdown of other behavior required to complete the procedure. Trainers can help alleviate anxiety by training a signal that indicates a needle stick or touch is about to happen. This helps clearly communicate to the animal when to expect contact (Video 3 online at www.vetexotic.theclinics.com).

Latency is a term used to describe slow or late presentation of a behavior after an animal has been given a cue. Latent performance of behavior is something that is often inadvertently created by the trainer. The following is a list of ways trainers create latency.

- Cueing repeatedly when the animal does not respond
- Asking for more behavior in the shaping process before the "quick response" criterion is met
- Not fading out showing reinforcers
- Cueing when the animal is not ready
- Cueing when it will be difficult for the animal to present the behavior
- Training when motivation for reinforcers is low
- Attempting to reduce slow presentation of behavior by withholding reinforcers

Trainers can prevent latent performance of behavior by using the following strategies when training a behavior:

- Train without distractions in the initial stages.
- Train when the animal is highly motivated for the reinforcers.
- Use high value reinforcers initially, then switch to using a variety of reinforcers once the behavior is fluent.
- Allow several seconds for the animal to respond to the cue. No response results in the removal of the opportunity to present the behavior and earn the reinforcer. This time out from positive reinforcement should only last a few seconds. This is followed by another opportunity for the animal to present the behavior with quick response to the cue.
- Cue the animal when it is highly likely to respond to the cue immediately. This allows trainers to reinforce presentation of the behavior paired with quick response.
- As the animal shows consistent immediate response to the cue, increase the criteria (attempt in new environments, with distractions, etc).[5]

CAPTURING BEHAVIOR

Because of the intricacies often involved in medical procedures, most behaviors trained for veterinary care are created by shaping with approximations. However, some behaviors are captured. Rather than breaking a goal behavior into steps or approximations to reinforce, trainers wait for the animal to present the action and reinforce.

Trainers can increase the likelihood the animal may present the behavior by arranging the environment. For example, if a trainer would like to train an animal to urinate on cue, they may place the scent or urine of another animal in the enclosure to encourage marking. When the animal urinates in response to the introduced scent the trainer reinforces. The trainer will then need to reset the environment or wait for another opportunity to reinforce the behavior. After the behavior has been reinforced repeatedly, the animal can associate earning reinforcers for doing the behavior and will begin to offer the behavior. A cue can be inserted as described previously (**Fig. 2**).

Capturing behavior presents several challenges. One is that the trainer must wait for presentation of the behavior. This may mean a great deal of time passes between opportunities to reinforce. If an animal only presents the behavior a few times in a day, it means it will take longer to build up enough reinforcement history for the animal to learn the action earns reinforcers.

If the behavior breaks down and is no longer presented on cue by the animal, the trainer is not able to relax criteria and quickly rebuild the behavior as can be done

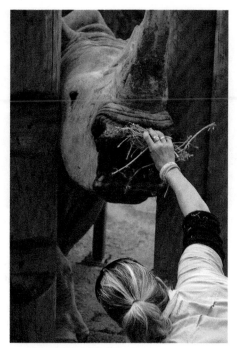

Fig. 2. A white rhinoceros (Ceratotherium simum) at the Auckland Zoo in New Zealand opens its mouth in anticipation of receiving food. This gives the trainer, Kathryn McKee, the opportunity to capture behavior rather than shape it with approximations.

when a behavior is shaped with approximations. Instead, the trainer will need to repeat the process of capturing the behavior.

TRAINING SESSION DYNAMICS

Effective animal trainers aim for creating an environment in which the animal will likely be receptive to a training session. This requires careful attention to a number of different elements. A primary concern for trainers is that the animal shows body language that indicates it is relaxed and comfortable in the designated training area. Allowing animals time to desensitize to the location, props, and people in the training area is a common practice in professional animal training. For some animals, this may take a few minutes. For others, it may require several sessions. An animal that is relaxed and comfortable is more likely to respond to the items made available as reinforcers for desired behavior.

Motivation for the potential reinforcers is also essential to an effective training session. Training sessions can be scheduled to coincide with times of the day when an animal may be most receptive to reinforcers, such as just before mealtime or when animals are most active (later in the day for crepuscular animals or first thing in the morning for diurnal animals).

Because positive reinforcement training involves access to desired reinforcers, animals can show anticipatory behaviors as they wait for a session to begin. To avoid creating a level of anxiety, it is helpful to arrange your training area before bringing the animal into the environment. Be prepared to train once the animal has desensitized to the environment (**Fig. 3**).

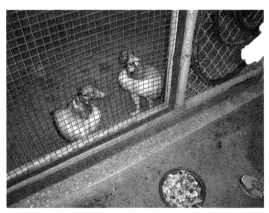

Fig. 3. Placing food in front of animal that cannot access it before a training session can create anxiety.

Trainers identify behaviors to train and steps or approximations that will be used to train each behavior before initiating a training session. To facilitate clear communication and faster training, it is also important to train one behavior at a time.

Once a session is started, it is important to remain focused on the animal until the session is terminated. Stopping and starting to gather supplies or re-stock reinforcers interrupts the session and can cause a loss of momentum. The session may require back tracking in approximations and rebuilding to the point at which the interruption occurred.

Prepare for a training session by doing the following:

- Desensitize animals to the environment, props, and/or people.
- Train when the animal is receptive to identified reinforcers.
- Arrange props before bringing animal to training area.
- Stock up on all training supplies and have them readily available before bringing animal to training area.
- Identify behaviors to train and approximations before starting session.
- Plan to train one behavior at a time.

Training sessions can vary in length depending on the animals' interest in the reinforcer. Training sessions last on average anywhere from 5 to 20 minutes. However, it is not unheard of to have shorter or longer sessions.

In general, the ideal session is one in which the animal is presenting behavior, focused on the task and/or trainer, and motivated for the reinforcers. This level of participation is usually what dictates the length of the session. As the animal becomes satiated on the reinforcer or if focus is lost due to environmental distractions, it is advantageous to end the training session. Latent performance of behavior is one undesired result of training under such circumstances.

Some session lengths are dictated by the amount of reinforcers available for training. Items may be limited for health or nutritional reasons.

A session may terminate for different reasons. Some trainers prefer to end a session before the animal shows less motivation for the reinforcers. Some prefer ending the session after the animal presents the behavior or an approximation of the behavior that is considered executed well. In these situations, trainers may offer more or highly preferred reinforcers to indicate the behavior presented was highly desired by the trainer. This use of behavior economics is also helpful when an animal presents a behavior that involves a high level of difficulty or effort by the animal. More work or more difficult action earns more or preferred reinforcers.

Other sessions may be interrupted by environmental distractions. In these situations, some animals are unable to redirect focus back to the training session. In these cases, going back and asking for a smaller approximation may help the animal refocus. However, in some cases, this is not possible, and rather than attempt to train, a common choice is to end the session and attempt training later.

Some trainers employ the use of a signal to indicate to the animal the training session is terminated and that reinforcers are no longer available. This is called an "end-of-session signal." Some trainers use a hand signal or show their hands are empty to indicate the end of a session. However, end-of-session signals can sometimes lead to undesired behaviors such as aggressive behavior, attempts to prevent trainers from leaving, and miscommunication to the animal.[3(pp358–360)] Many animals recognize the trainer gathering tools and reinforcers or walking away as an end-of-session signal. Other animals may be returned to their enclosure as indication the training session has terminated.

The time required to train a behavior will be dependent on the animal's level of comfort in the environment and with the trainer, familiarity with the training process, and the proficiency of the trainer. It will also be dependent on the animal's interest in the reinforcer. For animals that are comfortable and relaxed and motivated for reinforcers, it is often possible to train simple behaviors in 1 or 2 sessions. Some behaviors that are often easily trained in birds and small exotic mammals include targeting, getting on a scale, and accepting fluids from a syringe in preparation for training to accept oral medication (Video 4 online at www.vetexotic.theclinics.com).

Training sessions offer opportunities to reinforce desired behavior. More sessions can lead to learning the goal behavior quickly as long as the animal is motivated to participate. For some animals this may mean having several training sessions a day. If there is no urgency for training the behavior, sessions can be less frequent. The behavior goal may take longer to attain as the sessions will be spread out over more days. Once trained, most behaviors can be maintained by asking the animal to present the behavior weekly or monthly.

REINFORCERS AND MOTIVATION

The nature of positive reinforcement training is that presenting behaviors earns desired consequences for the animal. If these consequences serve to increase or maintain the behavior, they are considered reinforcers. Reinforcers can be many things. This can include food, touch, access to enrichment items, access to companions, etc (Video 5 online at www.vetexotic.theclinics.com).

Typically, animal training relies heavily on the use of primary reinforcers, usually food, to increase desired behavior. Food is an extremely effective reinforcer under certain conditions. It has also been shown that given the choice to use their adaptations to acquire food, animals will choose to do so. This is known as contra-freeloading.[6]

Food also allows for quick repetition of behavior. It is useful if the list of nonfood reinforcers is small or nonexistent. Food can also be paired with other items to expand the list nonfood reinforcers. It can help trainers avoid the use of negative reinforcement to increase behavior when applied well.[7] There are many benefits to using food as a reinforce (**Fig. 4**).

Most trainers initiate a training session by assessing the animal's interest in the reinforcer that is available. The level of interest will determine whether to continue with a training session at that time. To better gauge acceptable levels of motivation,

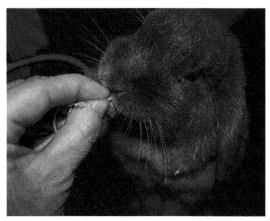

Fig. 4. The food reinforcers for a rabbit can include portions of the daily rations of greens and other produce.

trainers define a range of observable behaviors that can be matched with levels of motivation for reinforcers. For example, when a pine nut is offered to a macaw in a training scenario in which the bird is relaxed and comfortable and being asked to do nothing but accept food, the observations listed in **Table 2** could be used to rate motivation. For most situations, a medium level of interest in food reinforcers is sufficient to create desired responses. Working with an animal with a low level of interest in the reinforcer can create training problems such as slow response to the cue. Excessive levels of motivation often can result in less learning as the animal is too focused on trying to acquire food. Both extremes are not ideal for animal training.[8]

Table 2	
Assessing interest in reinforcers; in this example, a macaw is offered a pine nut	
Observed Behaviors	**Level of Motivation**
Holds pine nut in foot	Low
Bites tiny pieces off of pine nut slowly	Low
Drops half of the nut	Low
Wipes beak on perch (feaking observed)	Low
Proceeds to preen after drops nut	Low
Holds pine nut in foot and brings to mouth quickly	Medium
Quickly breaks nut into 2 or 3 pieces and swallow pieces	Medium
Directs attention back to trainer once nut is consumed	Medium
Swallows nut immediately without breaking into pieces	High
Quickly directs attention to trainer once nut is consumed	High
Offers trained behaviors in rapid succession	High
Presents behaviors equated with frustration or anxiety about food: may redirect aggressive behavior on nearby objects, birds, or people, stereotypic pacing, etc	Excessive
Aggressive behavior presented toward other birds if competing for the same food resource	Excessive

In the event the animal is not interested in food as a reinforce, there are a number of strategies trainers use to create motivation for food without the misuse of deprivation. For example, animals can be trained immediately preceding normal meal times, meal times can be staggered throughout the day to increase training opportunities, base diets can be provided at all times while preferred foods are saved for reinforcers to be offered during training, small pieces of food can be offered to allow for more repetitions before satiation, and/or the animal's regular diet can be offered during training only.[7] If any reduction in food provided is considered at all, the period is short lived. Once the learning has occurred, diets are quickly returned to levels considered typical for the animal. This has also been applied to human learners.[1(p220)] There are many examples in which the listed strategies for managing the delivery of food have proved to be successful in creating motivation for food reinforcers without compromising the health and welfare of the animal.

When training a new behavior, it is generally advised to use the most preferred reinforcer. Once the behavior has transitioned to maintenance, it can be advantageous to include other reinforcers. This can include a mix of food and nonfood reinforcers. This variety and unpredictability of what reinforcer will be offered can serve to maintain motivation for the animal to present the behavior.

Motivation for reinforcers can be influenced by many conditions, including the environment. An important goal is for the animal to be relaxed and comfortable in the training area. For example, an animal that prefers to be in enclosed areas such as a rat or guinea pig may quickly climb onto a scale if a shelter is provided on the scale. An overturned box with an access hole or hut on the scale can be tared out before the animal enters the shelter (Video 6 online at www.vetexotic.theclinics.com).

Other animals may respond with a higher level of comfort if a preferred companion is also in the training area. Some parrots and small mammals show behaviors indicative of discomfort when separated from conspecifics. The companion animal can be reinforced for remaining calm in the training area while the target animal is trained. Careful attention to arranging the environment to increase the comfort level of the animal in training will make it more likely the animal will respond to available reinforcers.

Trainers also aim for making it as easy as possible for the animal to present the behavior and acquire the reinforcer. For example, any behavior in which the animal must physically move more to do the action increases the difficulty. This means the animal must have higher motivation for the reinforcers provided. If the action is easier accomplished by moving or adjusting props, it will require less motivation. For example, training a parrot to climb over the lip of a crate to walk into it is more difficult than walking directly into the transport container that is flush with the surface upon which the bird is standing (**Fig. 5**).

Other factors that facilitate training are ensuring props are stationary and sufficient to hold the weight of the animal. When animals attempt to interact with a prop that moves, it can often create a fear response. This means perches, tables, scales, crates, etc, should remain motionless in initial stages of training. Overtime movement can be included if that is needed for the behavior goal. However, it should be considered another criterion to add to the shaping plan and trained accordingly.

BODY LANGUAGE

Trainers communicate to animals using the tools described in this article. Animals communicate using body language. It is therefore important for trainers to become familiar with the body language of the species identified for training.

The goal in animal training is for the animal to present body language that indicates comfort. Trainers are vigilant to avoid creating fear responses and aggressive

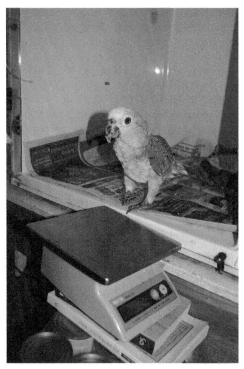

Fig. 5. Placing the scale so that is flush with the floor and steady makes it more likely a parrot will step onto it.

behavior. This requires trainers to practice excellent observational skills. It also requires trainers respond to body language immediately and appropriately. For example, if a trainer attempts to introduce a stethoscope to a parrot perched on a hand, if the bird looks for an escape path or leans slightly away, the trainer should respond by moving the stethoscope away from the animal in an effort to help the bird return to calm body language. The information learned in those moments tells the trainer that smaller approximations are required.

It is important for trainers to respond to the slightest indication of discomfort. This helps prevents animals from having to escalate their responses in order to cause circumstances they consider aversive to cease. Many animals learn to resort to aggressive behaviors, such as biting, when subtle body language fails.

Trainers also aim to avoid creating circumstances in which the animals fails to succeed in the training process and may present undesired behaviors such as self-injurious behaviors or redirecting aggressive behaviors. These actions, which might be labeled as frustration, can be the result of asking for approximations that are too big for the animal at that time. Sensitivity to animal body language will help trainers avoid this situation.

Approaching an animal for the first time is one of the most critical moments in animal training. The animal has no history with the trainer. The trainer has an opportunity to develop a relationship with the animal based on desired consequences. It is helpful to remain at a distance from an animal until it is possible to offer known desired reinforcers such as preferred food items. The trainer can show the animal he or she has food. The animal's body language will indicate whether it has an interest in the food. The animal may lean forward or take a step toward the trainer. The trainer may carefully move closer to allow the animal to accept the food. Again, the trainer will observe body language before moving closer or offering more food. If the animal shows sufficient interest in the food offered, training continues. Imposing oneself on an animal that is not receptive can cause the trainer to be considered an aversive as opposed to a source for desired reinforcers. Trainers who are aware of how their actions influence animal behavior and adjust to make the animal most comfortable typically excel at training animals to successfully cooperate in their own medical care.

OVERCOMING FEAR RESPONSES

Many medical behaviors involve objects, situations, or people that are unfamiliar to the animal. This can create a fear response if an animal is given no choice but to tolerate their presence. Unfortunately, this can create significant setbacks in the training process.

It is very important to avoid creating fear responses in successful animal training for medical behaviors. Systematic desensitization is usually the first step in preventing a fear response. For example, if the goal is for a rabbit to accept medication from a syringe and the rabbit has no known history with syringes, the object can be placed at a distance from the animal. The goal is for the presence of the object to be noticed by the rabbit, and at the same time the rabbit's body language remains calm and relaxed. As long as this criterion is maintained, the syringe can be moved closer to the animal. The rabbit may not interact with the object but via this process will be calm in the presence of the object.

Systematic desensitization is an excellent process for introducing many objects commonly used in medical procedures such as stethoscopes, syringes, scales, swabs, towels, etc. They often can be left outside the enclosure and gradually moved closer over time. Once comfortable with the presence of the object, shaping with approximations can be used to train the animal to interact with the object.

In addition to systematic desensitization, trainers will also find value in pairing known reinforcers with the presence of objects or circumstances that can potentially trigger fear responses. For example, offering preferred food items when a veterinary professional is present can increase the value of the presence of the person to the animal. Eventually, the veterinary professional can offer the preferred food item. Pairing this process with the avoidance of creating fear responses and empowering the animal to choose to participate are critical components in teaching animals to cooperate in their own medical care (**Fig. 6**).

GENERALIZATION OF BEHAVIORS

A common complaint is that the animal will do the desired behavior at home but not at the veterinary clinic. This is because additional training is required for a behavior to be fluent under other circumstances in addition to the one in which it was trained. This procedure is called *generalization.* Typically to generalize behavior, trainers retrain the behavior under different conditions. This may include different locations, with different trainers, with slightly different props, etc.

Each change in condition is new criterion added to the process. This may require the trainer to relax other criteria and rebuild the behavior using the shaping procedure. The goal is to repeat the process under enough different conditions that the environment or other changes no longer create a distraction. The animal remains focused on the task at hand despite the surroundings. This is critical for medical behaviors that require the animal to cooperate in new environments. If the behavior is generalized, the new circumstances will not present a problem.

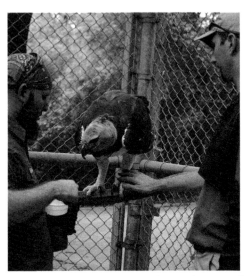

Fig. 6. Touching the foot of a Harpy eagle (Harpia harpyja) is paired with the delivery of preferred food items.

It is helpful to keep as many aspects of the behavior or procedure as consistent as possible to increase the likelihood the animal will succeed under the new condition, such as by using the same tools, props, or trainers when possible.

SUMMARY

Training animals to cooperate in their own medical care is fast becoming common practice in animal facilities such as zoos and laboratories. It is gradually crossing over into the companion animal world. As growing numbers of veterinary professionals learn the value of this science based training technology and how to apply it, more animals will benefit from stress free medical care. Supporting the positive reinforcement animal training movement and understanding the application of science-based training technology are important steps toward improving the health and welfare of the animals we steward.

SUPPLEMENTARY DATA

Supplementary data related to this article can be found online at doi:10.1016/j.cvex.2012.06.006.

REFERENCES

1. Sidman M. Coercion and its fallout. Boston (MA): Authors Cooperative; 1989. p. 80, 119, 186.
2. Chance P. First course in applied behavior analysis. Pacific Grove (CA): Brooks Cole; 1998. p. 462.
3. Ramirez K. Husbandry. Animal training: successful animal management through positive reinforcement. Chicago (IL): Shedd Aquarium Press; 1999. p. 15.
4. Mazur J. Predicting the strength of a conditioned reinforcer. Effects of delay and uncertainty. Curr Dir Psychol Sci 1993;2:70–4.

5. Heidenreich BE. Latent performance of behavior. How to train quick response to the cue. In: Proceedings International Association of Avian Trainers and Educators Conference: Nashville, February 15–18, 2006.
6. Jensen GD. Preference for bar pressing over 'freeloading' as a function of number of rewarded presses. J Exp Psychol 1963;65:451–4.
7. Heidenreich BE. Managing the deliverance of food to create motivation. In: Proceedings Mid-Atlantic States Association of Avian Veterinarians: Virginia Beach, April 2–4, 2006.
8. Heidenreich BE. The ethics of animal training and handling. Presented at The Proceedings International Association of Avian Trainers and Educators Conference: Alphen aan den Rijn, The Netherlands, March 5–8, 2008.

Animal Learning and Training
Implications for Animal Welfare

Sabrina I.C.A. Brando, BSc

KEYWORDS

- Animal welfare • Learning • Training • Positive reinforcement

KEY POINTS

- A definition of animal welfare is the state of the individual as it attempts to cope with its environment.
- Welfare concerns all of the mechanisms for coping, involving physiology, behavior, feelings, and pathologic responses.
- When training programs are not in place the animal's welfare could be impaired.
- Some of the behaviors an animal exhibits can be used to gain insight into how the animal feels about the environment, caretakers, and procedures.
- Many contemporary animal trainers and care specialists focus on building relationships using positive reinforcement.

ANIMAL WELFARE

The field of animal welfare is rapidly evolving and growing. Green and Mellor[1] write "The literature on animal welfare is diverse and expanding and reveals that ideas about animal welfare have evolved since it became established as a field of scientific investigations about 25–30 years ago.[2–4] Its scientific roots are multi-disciplinary[5] and include fields such as ethology, physiology, pathology, biochemistry, genetics, immunology, immunology, cognitive neural science and veterinary epidemiology.[3,4,6] In addition, scientific thinking about animal welfare has been influenced by societal views on what constitutes acceptable and unacceptable ways of treating animals, views which reflected prevailing and evolving ethical, social, cultural, religious, economic and other values."[3,7,8] In the assessment of animal welfare previously there was a focus on pain, stress, maladaptive behavior, and disease; the focus was on reducing negative animal welfare states. Now the assessment of animal welfare also includes positive welfare states, the presence of feelings of pleasure or contentment; the assessment is based the holistic approach of "considering the whole animal."[9] Mendl

The author has nothing to disclose.
AnimalConcepts, Zoom 1813, 8225 KM, Lelystad, The Netherlands
E-mail address: sbrando@animalconcepts.eu

and colleagues[10] write "Concerns for animal welfare are generally based on the assumption that non-human animals can subjectively experience emotional (affective) states and hence can suffer or experience pleasure."[11–14]

Broom[15] writes "Health is part of welfare and it refers to what is happening in body systems, including those in the brain, which combat pathogens, tissue damage or physiologic disorder. Health is the state of an individual as it attempts to cope with pathology. With disease challenges, as well as with other challenges, difficult or inadequate adaptation results in poor welfare." "Poor welfare is often associated with lack of control over interactions with the environment of the individual, ie, with difficulty in adapting. To use animals in a human-orientated environment, and to ensure that the welfare of those animals is good, we need to know about the abilities of animals to adapt. At the individual level, adaptation is the use of regulatory systems, with their behavioral and physiologic components, to help an individual to cope with its environmental conditions."[16] Broom[17] also writes "A definition of animal welfare is: the state of the individual as it attempts to cope with its environment. Welfare concerns all of the mechanisms for coping: involving physiology, behavior, feelings and pathologic responses. Welfare is a wider term than health but health is an important part of welfare. Animal welfare is a scientific concept that describes a potentially measurable quality of a living animal at a particular time. Behavioral measures are also of particular value in welfare assessment. The fact that an animal avoids an object or event, strongly gives information about its feelings and hence about its welfare. The stronger the avoidance the worse the welfare while the object is present or the event is occurring."

To ensure high welfare levels for animals, caretakers need to analyze and evaluate the methods used to achieve desired behavior, to understand how learning affects their welfare **Table 1**. Caretakers can use behavioral observations together with physiologic observations as tools to gain insight into how animals experience their environment, staff members, and conspecifics. Caretakers can determine what matters to animals in their care and what are their welfare needs.[10,18] In regard to medical care many animals experience situations considered to be associated with negative welfare states, such as lack of control over environment, lack of choices, fear responses, coercion, and exposure to aversives.

In some cases choosing a negative welfare state is most conducive to supporting health care. For example, an animal may need movement to be limited to ensure healing. However, other commonly experienced procedures have the potential to be modified to promote positive welfare states. For example, routine capture and restraint can be trained using positive reinforcement so that an animal voluntarily participates in the procedure. Health is part of welfare; however, in practice the emphasis is often on

Table 1
Welfare indicators

Positive Welfare Indicators	Negative Welfare Indicators
Interest in activities or enrichment	Body damage
Behaviors indicative of comfort or rest	Apathy
Play behaviors	Self-mutilation
Acceptable interactions with caretakers	Learned helplessness
Physical and psychological fitness	High vigilance
Normal sleep patterns	Stereotypic behaviors
Normal grooming and bathing behaviors	Little to no control over the environment
Normal interactions with conspecifics	Extensive huddling or hiding from caretakers
Control and choice over the environment	

health, and often only on physical health. By focusing on welfare, including physical and psychological health, caregivers can provide optimal care for the animals they steward.

LEARNING IS ALWAYS OCCURRING

Animals are learning all the time. They are learning about routine procedures, such as shifting, weighing, and nail clipping. They are also aware of and learning about the frequency, quantity, and time of feeding; cleaning; care staff personalities; show times; and enrichment activities. Because animals are constantly learning, albeit through different mechanisms, animals are almost always "in training." They learn about the environment, housing conditions, social dynamics, when the areas are cleaned, and when animals will be handled. The animals might learn about shifting, handling, or weighing but not necessarily participate in these procedures on a voluntary basis. When medical, behavior and other care programs are not actively and extensively discussed, planned, and analyzed many things can lead to poor welfare. When animals are not trained to voluntarily participate in their care (to shift into areas, to be on scales, to feel comfortable being handled or when treated) the procedures and outcomes for these animals are often aversive in nature. Water sprays, brooms, stones, loud noises, the threatening posture of a human body, grabbing hands, and nets and gloves have all been used in a coercive manner to move animals; to handle; and to control and restrain animals for husbandry and medical procedures (personal observations).

LACK OF A TRAINING PROGRAM AFFECTS WELFARE

When training programs are not in place animal welfare suffers. For example, access to food is often misused or abused when animals are not trained to voluntarily shift into holding areas. The food is positioned to encourage animals to move to desired areas, such as dens or crates for handling and medical examination. If animals show fear responses to those areas they either have to enter to eat or go without food. This severely reduces the animal's choices and control over access to food. This often results in pacing, spending excessive amounts of time close to shift doors, or other maladaptive behaviors. The animal may be motivated to eat but will not dare to enter the area because of past experiences of being trapped or captured. If the animal is very hungry then it might run in quickly to access food and immediately exit again. Many animals wait for the caretakers to leave. Caretakers will observe the food is gone when they return. Some animals spend a considerable amount of time in off exhibit holding areas when caretakers are not around (observed by cameras). These animals have learned that capture depends on staff being present. Sometimes animals need to be enclosed inside for enclosure repair, cleaning, or medical examinations. In these situations some caretakers wait long periods of time for the animal to enter the holding area. When the animal finally comes in, the door is shut behind them. This often results in pacing, escape behaviors, or huddling behavior (depending on the individual and species) until the door is opened again and the animal can run out. Most animal care staff and veterinarians confirm that one trial learning is often sufficient for the animal to learn to stay away from those areas or people involved in the capture for considerable amounts of time afterward.

The behaviors an animal exhibits can be used to gain insight into how the animal feels about the environment, the caretakers, and the procedures. Pacing, huddling together, alarm calls, hiding when a person shows up, and not approaching caretakers or veterinarians are all examples of animals that are experiencing reduced welfare. These behaviors should be used as an indicator that the behavior and care program is not functioning at best practice levels and that changes need to be made to reduce fear and anxiety toward humans, procedures, and the environment.

ANIMAL RESPONSE TO HEALTH CARE

The accounts of animals identifying veterinarians from the crowd, even when dressed up to look like a caretaker or technician, are many. Because of busy schedules many veterinarians do not have time to spend feeding animals, playing with them, or offering enrichment. One of the reasons some veterinary procedures, such as blood sampling, are sometimes transferred to zoo keepers is that often as soon as the veterinarian comes into sight, animals run away, hide, or are no longer cooperative. The animals have learned to associate the veterinarian with unpleasant procedures, anxiety, or pain. The animals often never see the veterinarian outside of these medical procedures, resulting in an association based only on aversives. Animals are often asked to shift into holding areas or crates before the veterinarian arrives to increase the chances of success for the medical examination. Caretakers need to consider that this might facilitate getting the procedure accomplished in the short term but may make shifting for future examinations more difficult. When an animal shifts into a holding area and it is followed-up with aversive experiences, a decrease in the success rate of these behaviors is observed.

Some veterinarians are able to find time to interact with animals and build a trusting relationship. These animals learn to associate the veterinarian with pleasant activities, such as feeding, resting, and playing. Something unpleasant rarely happens, and when it does the event is signaled. For example the word "door" can be used to signal when a door opens or shuts, and can then be anticipated by the animal. This reduces high vigilance and makes it more likely the animal will be inclined to participate in species-specific behaviors, social activities, grooming, eating, and so forth.

In the best scenario the animal participates voluntarily in its own care. Unless animals are in rehabilitation and reintroduction programs with special requirements, all animals housed in captivity should not have to live with fear and anxiety toward humans or their environment. How the animal responds to its environment and the way it copes with negative and positive stressors is important for understanding the individual animal's welfare. Not teaching animals to be comfortably handled can result in fear, anxiety, or aggressive behavior. Aggressive behavior often leads to the animal being moved on to another collection, into shelters, or at times euthanasia. Furthermore, many people do not like working with animals that present aggressive behavior or fear responses. This could result in less motivation to provide optimal care for such individuals.

Understanding how different learning mechanisms work can help reduce unnecessary fear, anxiety, extreme vigilance, aggressive behavior, and program-induced stereotypic or other undesired behaviors. This can greatly improve their welfare and the experiences of positive welfare states and reduce the negative experiences often related to involuntary procedures and circumstances.

CHANGES IN ANIMAL TRAINING

Understanding animal learning is an important facet of being an animal care specialist. This applies to veterinarians, curators, zookeepers, and pet owners. Because animals are constantly learning caretakers need to be aware of the effects of their decisions, attitudes, and actions. Veterinarians encounter a great number of animals with behavioral problems. This is observed in companion animals and captive wild animals. Because of this there is a growing need for more and more veterinarians who have an interest in specializing in animal behavior and learning.

The field of animal training has seen beneficial changes. These changes include a transition to the use of methods that focus on positive reinforcement and heightened sensitivity to the animal's body language to avoid creating fear responses and aggressive behaviors. There has been a shift away from coercive methods of training and an emphasis on empowering the animal. This has led to good relationships with animals based on trust. Positive reinforcement has been applied to species varying from mammals and reptiles to birds and fish.[19–23]

Many animal species are trained in a free-contact scenario. The trainer and the animal have full access to one another. In this situation the use of aversives can lead to dangerous situations, particularly when working in close proximity to an animal.[19] Acceptable ways of animal training have been under discussion for many years, especially in the dog training world. Yin writes about the dominance controversy[24]: "Virtually everyone who started as a dog trainer over 15–20 years ago started out using traditional dog training techniques: similar to those used by Cesar Millan (National Geographic's The Dog Whisperer). This is how most dogs were trained back then. As a result we have first-hand experience as to why and when such punishment-based techniques might work, the pitfalls, and why and when other techniques work better. Traditional training techniques are based on the idea that we must become the dominant leader and rule our pets the way a wolf would rule a pack." Many dog trainer associations have opposed traditional dog training methods, and in February 2009 the American Veterinary Society of Animal Behavior has also opposed these punitive methods. The American Veterinary Society of Animal Behavior issued a position statement about the use of punishment for behavior modification in animals, detailing nine possible adverse effects of using punishment when training dogs.[25] Training methods with frequent use of punishers and other aversive methods should be modified by reducing or abolishing the use of punishers in facilities, veterinary clinics, and at home. Punishers do not inform the animal what it is that we would like her or him to do, only what was the incorrect response. The frequent use of punishers can also instill anxiety in regard to learning. Animals may hesitate to respond in fear of making the wrong decision. This response can become slower until the animal may choose not to respond at all.

Focusing on positive reinforcement training allows the caregiver to build trust and a bond with the animals, while at the same time promoting the desired behaviors and creating a stimulating, interesting, and safe learning environment. In traditional animal training many practices that result in poor animal welfare have been used. For example, excessive food deprivation has often been used to motivate the animals. In other cases, gregarious animals were placed in social isolation and received limited human contact because of undesired behavior (personal observations). Many things are done to animals, including grabbing, poking, squeezing, spraying with water hoses, and scaring with loud noises because there is a perceived need to control the animal. Humans have also practiced these methods on animals because they can. This is because often the animals are small enough to be overpowered and handled, or in an enclosure where they can easily be accessed. If the animal could potentially harm a human and there were no protective barriers, it is unlikely a caretaker would think of waving food in front of an animal to gain cooperation and then put it back in the container. If the animal could potentially harm a human and there were no barriers, it is unlikely a caretaker would think of using the spray of water from a hose or throwing stones to get an animal to move to other areas. Most humans would never grab or hold an animal down if it was thought the animal could hurt or kill the handler (except perhaps in a medical emergency). The reasons things have traditionally been done this way are many: because humans have been able to get away with such practices, often because of time constraints, the perceived ease of using such methods, "because we have always done it this way," or just because the alternative options have not yet been considered.

Many contemporary animal trainers and care specialists focus on building relationships using positive reinforcement. They are not only concerned with the correct application of behavioral learning principles but they also pay attention to and consider the effect of human body language, posture, and communication of the animals in their care.[26]

UNDERSTANDING PRINCIPLES OF LEARNING

Although there are many processes through which animals can learn, this article focuses mainly on classical and operant conditioning with an emphasis on positive reinforcement as it applies to daily husbandry and medical care procedures. "Classical conditioning is a process of behavior modification in which a subject learns to respond in a desired manner such that a neutral stimulus is repeatedly presented in association with a stimulus (the unconditioned stimulus) that elicits a natural response (the unconditioned response) until the neutral stimulus alone elicits the same response (now called the conditioned response). For example, in Pavlov's experiments, food is the unconditioned stimulus that produces salivation, a reflex or unconditioned response. The bell is the conditioned stimulus, which eventually produces salivation in the absence of food. This salivation is the conditioned response."[27]

In a veterinary example an ophthalmoscope used to investigate the eyes of an animal and a bottle of eye drops are the unconditioned stimuli. The bright light used with the ophthalmoscope and drops applied to the eyes make the rat close its eyes (unconditioned response). Over time the bright light becomes associated with the ophthalmoscope and the drops become associated with the bottle. Eventually the presence of the ophthalmoscope or the bottle can elicit closing of the eyes as if the light or the drops were there (conditioned response). In this example the animal may start to squint when the veterinarian picks up the ophthalmoscope or bottle of eye drops. These at first unconditioned stimuli became conditioned stimuli, eliciting the same response (squinting or closing of the eyes) as if the bright light or the drops where there. Classical conditioning has taken place when such reactions are observed. In this example it is important to note that although training may not have been intentionally occurring the animal has learned a specific response to the stimuli. In addition to the resulting behavior, there are also underlying emotional states associated with the process, such as fear, anxiety, or pleasure. Veterinary professionals who are aware of how their actions influence animal behavior and emotional states are better prepared to improve welfare states in regard to medical procedures.

This also applies to other principles of learning. Understanding how positive and negative reinforcement, and positive and negative punishment are used to influence behavior can make a veterinary professional more cognizant of his or her actions. Learning processes in which an aversive is applied to decrease behavior (positive punishment) or removed to increase behavior (negative reinforcement) are generally considered options only when less intrusive choices (positive reinforcement and negative punishment) are not successful. The animal training community has shown that positive reinforcement can be used successfully for voluntary participation in medical procedures in several species. Some examples include training animals to cooperate in nail clipping, crate training, blood sampling, radiographs, and accepting oral medications. Positive reinforcement trainers are highly aware of aversives experiences and how they affect behavior and the relationship between the trainer and the animal and therefore rarely consider the use of aversives as an option in training. This same sensitivity applied in the veterinary setting can lead to more successful medical procedures with little or no stress. For additional information see the articles on the application of science-based training technology and a framework for solving behavior problems elsewhere in this issue.

To better understand what learning principles are in play veterinary professionals need to identify if a behavior has been increased, maintained, or decreased. They also need to identify what consequences resulted from the presentation of the observed behavior. Was an aversive removed? Was an item of value (eg, a preferred food item) presented and consumed? Careful scrutiny of behavior change and the process help veterinary professionals refine practices and focus on the use of positive reinforcement–based methods

Not understanding and recognizing these principles can have serious impact on the care and welfare of animals. Animals that learn fear responses and aggressive behavior toward humans because of heavy-handed treatment procedures may be difficult or dangerous to treat. These patterns can be broken by understanding how the learning process works and adjusting handling strategies to train the patient to cooperate voluntarily. Cooperation can make medical care easier, and it can also influence emotional states. Understanding and recognizing positive and negative welfare, and matching behavior to internal states, is essential to improve animal welfare.

Animal trainers are also careful to observe the animals they work with and keep track of changes in behavior, preferences, and learning. Changes can occur depending on such variables as life stages, seasons, the weather, pain, and social dynamics, which can work alone or together. Good trainers adapt when necessary, and are sensitive to the animal's needs. Good trainers also understand how the different mechanisms and tools work together or effects caused by incorrect application.

Ramirez proposes that "training is teaching."[28] By teaching animals to participate in their daily health and husbandry care the stress that is related to these procedures[29–34] can be significantly reduced. Positive reinforcement can be used to reduce fear responses and aggressive behavior. Positive reinforcement can be used to train animals to be cooperative in their care and provide a stimulating environment in which they can experience positive welfare states.

FEAR RESPONSES AND ANIMAL WELFARE

Reducing fear responses is important to animal welfare. Desensitization and counterconditioning are the tools of choice to address fear responses and provide positive welfare states. Stafford[35] writes "According to the training glossary of the International Marine Animal Trainers' Association (IMATA), desensitization is a "process of using time or experience to change an animal's perception of a stimulus from a value, ... to neutral or no value." When trainers think of desensitization, they are usually concerned with reducing the aversive value of a stimulus, such as eliminating a dog's fearful reactions to thunderstorms by providing reinforcing consequences for calm responses. However, it is important to remember that desensitization also cuts the other way. For example, leaving the same few dog toys out day after day can reduce the reinforcement value of those toys. Similarly, using a clicker repeatedly, tooting all day long on a whistle, or shouting "good boy" over and over again to mark precise behavior approximations (what the Breland's[36] first called "bridging a behavior") without following those signals with meaningful reinforcement can weaken (ie, desensitize) the effectiveness of those bridging stimuli. Because a strong bridge (in whatever form) is needed to accurately and precisely reward improvements in the behaviors one wants to teach, including reducing fearful and anxious responses, it is vital that one not inadvertently desensitize animals to this key training tool through its overuse and underreinforcement.

Counterconditioning is "pairing one stimulus that evokes one response with another that evokes an opposite response, so that the first stimulus comes to evoke the second response."[37] For example, if a dog is afraid of the nail clippers, the dog can be fed its favorite food as the veterinarian approaches with the nail clippers. "The goal is to replace the animal's apprehension with the pleasure elicited by the food. Counter conditioning must be done gradually, however; if the process is rushed, the favorite food may take on the fear association instead."[37] A clear video is available.[38]

By teaching animals to participate in their daily care they gain more control and choice over their environment. Caregivers can offer the animal the opportunity to participate and collaborate, rather than imposing procedures on them. This can decrease the fear and stress related to procedures and can also increase the motivation of animals to participate in pretrained procedures. Concern for mental and physical well-being includes understanding learning principles and addressing fear responses, and can ultimately lead to an increase in the welfare standard of the animals in one's care.

THE HUMAN-ANIMAL RELATIONSHIP

"We should work with animals as if gates and doors weren't there; as if they could leave any moment they wanted. If they then decide to stay and be with you, then you can say you have a good bond and the animal is truly interested in being with you" (J. McBain, personal communication, 2008).

Veterinarians, curators, zookeepers, and pet owners are all "trainers." Whether aware of it or not, each is training the animals in their care, influencing behavior, and affecting the human-animal relationship. An animal can learn that a human's presence results in desired consequences or undesired consequences. This affects how an animal responds to each individual it encounters. This means the decisions made in regard to how medical care is provided can have consequences. Some consequences have lasting effect. Doing something to an animal that is unpleasant just one time, such as a short restraint procedure, can be enough to teach the animal to mistrust a handler for a long time. Although an emergency may require such action, it is important to consider or accept the consequences before proceeding. Best care practices require refining some of the traditional methods used to provide medical care. With the knowledge that many animals respond with fear or aggressive behavior to capture and restraint, at the very least animal care programs should include a strategy for reducing stress for these procedures either through training or arranging the environment so that the process is as stress-free as possible. Although it is possible to get animals to cooperate by other means, such as using positive punishment or other coercive methods, this does not result in good welfare states. It is important to attend to the animal's medical needs but the process with which it is done is equally important to maintaining a trusting relationship with the animal. Even when restricted for time, veterinary professionals have options. For example, not all restraint procedures require a strong hold for the duration of the treatment. Negative reinforcement in which the handler relaxes restraint when the animal is calm can teach the animal to present calm behavior during restraint procedures. These refinements can be incorporated readily, are easy for an animal to learn, and improve animal welfare when less intrusive options are not possible.

When working with animals it can be helpful to consider how the animal perceives the humans it encounters. This can be measured by looking at its behavioral responses toward humans. Does the animal orient toward people, move toward or away from people? Is the animal eager to participate in interactions with a human? How does the animal behave when people are absent? How does the animal respond to specific individuals? Does behavior change when certain individuals come or go? An animal that associates desired consequences with human presence is likely to seek interaction. This can be helpful to building cooperation in medical care.

However, it is also important for many species to be independent or maintain social dynamics with conspecifics. This means finding a balance between the reinforcing value of humans and other aspects of the animal's life. Technology, such as pressure plates, timers, and infrared sensors, are being used to create and automate enriching environments. Animal behavior can trigger desired consequences without the need for a trainer to be present or perceived. The implications for this are particularly important for those animals with strong fear responses or aggressive behavior toward humans or animals that may be destined for release in the wild. A paper dealing with choice and control opportunities in animal training and enrichment is in preparation to further explain this growing technology and its application. (Brando S. Choice and control opportunities in animal training and enrichment. Submitted for publication).

A trusting relationship can help facilitate animals to cooperate in their own medical care. Other key factors include providing an environment in which the animal is motivated to participate, is safe, and is enriched by the experience. It is also important to recognize when an animal does not want to participate. "To develop and maintain an animal's positive attitude toward learning....this means that the trainer cares about the overall learning experience of the animal...."[39] When an animal does not want to participate it is the trainer's responsibility to evaluate the situation. Rather than blaming the animal, the trainer looks into the factors that may be contributing to the lack of collaboration. This might include medical issues, discomfort with the environment, social dynamics, lack of interest in reinforcers, mistrust of staff members, or the particular situation. It is important to focus on positive methods and trust-building interactions, even in periods of noncooperation.

Building a trusting relationship with an animal may take time but it can have a positive impact on animal welfare.[40] It also requires consistency and clarity in behavior and signals used to communicate with animals. These signals include those that inform the animal about upcoming procedures or request participation in voluntary husbandry or medical behaviors. If handlers do not have the opportunity to train animals to enter a crate on a voluntary basis and have to resort to catching the animal on a regular basis, handlers may want to consider having a distinct signal for catching versus noncatching events. For example, an orange jumpsuit could signal a capture will take place; it might not fully reduce the anxiety during the capture events, but in the absence of the orange suit animals know that capture will not happen. This can help reduce anxiety toward caregivers outside the capture situations (personal observation).

"The development of these relationships is enriching to both personnel and animals inasmuch as people who care about their animals are committed to promoting and ensuring the well-being of those animals."[40,41] Staats and colleagues[42] propose that the "cognitive intent to act in ways directed toward the well-being" of the animal (which they define as commitment) has a significant role in the relationship that develops between a person and an animal." This commitment, the authors suggest, is measured by sustaining the relationship despite personal effort, time, money, and patience. This does not necessarily mean investing lots of time; sometimes just several minutes a day make a positive difference.[43]

Caregivers often expect a lot from an animal; go there, stay here, be calm, do not aggress, keep your mouth open, and so forth. Sometimes situations and environments are difficult. Animals might not always get or do what they want, go where they want, or be with whom they want, but they need to have some control over what happens to them. It is important to ask how much control and how many choices do the animals have in their day to day life. Caregivers who are serious about animal welfare and creating environments that promote positive welfare states need to ask and then act on these questions.

SUMMARY

Animals are always learning. An understanding of learning theories can help caregivers address, treat, and prevent many of the behavioral problems seen in captivity. Positive reinforcement training gives animal caretakers opportunities to teach animals to voluntarily participate in their care and to interact with their environment. Understanding how animals learn can allow caregivers to use such procedures as desensitization and counterconditioning to reduce fear and anxiety. This can lead to trusting relationships between caregiver and animal and allows for positive experiences for staff members and animals. Animal behavior and learning are important aspects of a holistic approach to animal welfare. An understanding of the role they play in animal welfare is fundamental to ensure that caregivers provide the best in animal care practices.

REFERENCES

1. Green TC, Mellor DJ. Extending ideas about animal welfare assessment to include 'quality of life' and related concepts. N Z Vet J 2011;59(6):263–71.
2. Nordenfelt L. Animal and human health and welfare: a comparative philosophical analysis. Wallingford (United Kingdom): CABI; 2006.
3. Fraser D. Understanding animal welfare: the science in its cultural context. Oxford (United Kingdom): Wiley-Blackwell; 2008.
4. Mellor OJ, Patterson-Kane E, Stafford KJ. Introduction to animal welfare. In: Sciences of animal welfare. Oxford (United Kingdom): Wiley-Blackwell; 2009. p. 3–94.
5. Sandoe P, Simonsen H. Assessing animal welfare: where does science end and philosophy begin? Anim Welfare 1992;1(4):257–67.
6. Lassen J, Sandoe P, Forkman B. Happy pigs are dirty! Conflicting perspectives on animal welfare. Livest Sci 2006;103:221–30.
7. Fraser D. Animal ethics and animal welfare science: bridging two cultures. Appl Anim Behav Sci 1999;65(17):1–89.
8. Fisher MW, Mellor OJ. Developing a systematic strategy incorporating ethical, animal welfare and practical principles to guide the genetic improvement of dairy cattle. N Z Vet J 2008;65:100–6.
9. Simonsen HB. Assessment of animal welfare by a holistic approach: behavior, health and measured opinion. Acta Agric Scand A Anim Sci 1996;27:91–6.
10. Mendl M, Burman OH, Parker RM, et al. Cognitive bias as an indicator of animal emotion and welfare: emerging evidence and underlying mechanisms. Appl Anim Behav Sci 2009;118:3–4, 161–81.
11. Dawkins MS. From an animal's point of view: motivation, fitness and animal welfare. Behav Brain Sci 1990;13:1–61.
12. Mendl M. Assessing the welfare state. Nature 2001;410:31–2.
13. Mendl M, Paul ES. Consciousness, emotion and animal welfare: insights from cognitive science. Anim Welfare 2004;13:S17–25.
14. Boissy A, Manteuffel G, Jensen MB, et al. Assessment of positive emotions in animals to improve their welfare. Physiol Behav 2007;92:375–97.

15. Broom DM. Coping, stress and welfare. In: Broom DM, editor. Coping with challenge: welfare in animals including humans. Berlin: Dahlem University Press; 2001. p. 1–9.
16. Broom DM. Behavior and welfare in relation to pathology. Appl Anim Behav Sci 2006;97:71–83.
17. Broom DM. A history of animal welfare science. Acta Biotheor 2011;59:121–37.
18. Wemelsfelder F. How animals communicate quality of life: the qualitative assessment of behavior. Anim Welfare 2007;16:25–31.
19. Turner TN, Tompkins C. Aggression: exploring the causes and possible reduction techniques. Soundings 1990;15:11–5.
20. Heidenreich B, Corredor E, Compton N. Harpy eagle training: exploring the potential of positive reinforcement. Presented at the International Association of Avian Trainers and Educators Conference: Albuquerque, New Mexico, March 3–6, 2010.
21. Heidenreich B. The ethics of animal training and handling. Presented at The International Association of Avian Trainers and Educators Conference: Alphen aan den Rijn, The Netherlands, March 5–8, 2008.
22. Kother G, Dempsey S. Enrichment and training in reptiles. Presented at the REEC 4th UK & Ireland REEC: Port Lympne and Howletts Wild Animal Parks, Aspinall Foundation, Kent, UK 13–16th 2012.
23. Christen DR, Schreiber CM. Stretcher training of a Giant Manta (*Manta birostris*) to facilitate physical examinations. Soundings 2010;35:2.
24. Yin S. The dominance controversy. Available at: http://drsophiayin.com/philosophy/dominance/?/dominance.php. Accessed May 26, 2012.
25. The American Veterinary Society of Animal Behavior AVSAB position statement the use of punishment for behavior modification in animals. Available at: http://www.avsabonline.org/avsabonline/images/stories/Position_Statements/Combined_Punishment_Statements.pdf. Accessed May 26, 2012.
26. Davis C, Harris G. Redefining our relationships with the animals we train: leadership and posture. Soundings 2006;31(4):6–8.
27. Classical conditioning definition. Available at: http://www.thefreedictionary.com/classical+conditioning. Accessed May 23, 2012.
28. Ramirez K. Animal training: successful animal management through positive reinforcement. Chicago: Shedd Aquarium Press; 1999.
29. Brando S. Advances in husbandry training in marine mammal care programs. Int J Comp Psychol 2010;23:777–91.
30. Desportes G, Buholzer L, Anderson-Hansen K, et al. Decrease stress; train your animals: the effect of handling methods on cortisol levels in harbor porpoises (*Phocoena phocoena*) under human care. Aquatic Mammals 2007;33:286–92.
31. Reinhardt V. Training adult male rhesus monkeys to actively cooperate during in-homecage venipuncture. Anim Tech 1991;42:11–7.
32. Heidenreich B. Training birds for husbandry and medical behavior to reduce or eliminate stress. Presented at the Association of Avian Veterinarians Conference: New Orleans, Louisiana, August 17–19, 2004.
33. McKinley J, Buchanan-Smith HM, Bassett L, et al. Training common marmosets (*Callithrix jacchus*) to cooperate during routine laboratory procedures: ease of training and time investment. J Appl Anim Welf Sci 2003;6:209–20.
34. Reinhardt V. Working with rather than against macaques during blood collection. J Appl Anim Welf Sci 2003;6:189–97.
35. Stafford G. Desensitization for life. Soundings 2011;36:2.
36. Bailey R, Gillaspy J. Operant psychology goes to the fair. Marian and Keller Breland in the popular press. 1947-1966. Behav Anal 2005;28:143–59.

37. Counter conditioning. Available at: http://www.clickertraining.com/glossary. Accessed May 26, 2012.

38. Yin S. Aggressive toenail trim. Available at: http://www.youtube.com/watch?v=WWZUcLfHXL. Accessed May 26, 2012.

39. Sullivan TJ. The yin and yang of positive reinforcement training. Soundings 2002; 27(2):28–30.

40. Bayne K. Development of the human-research animal bond and its impact on animal well-being. ILAR J 2002;43(1):4–9.

41. Davis H. How human/animal bonding affects the animals. In: Krulisch L, Mayer S, Simmonds RC, editors. The human\research animal relationship. Greenbelt (MD): Scientists Center for Animal Welfare; 1996. p. 67–75.

42. Staats S, Pierfelice L, Kim C, et al. A theoretical model for human health and the pet connection. J Am Vet Med Assoc 1999;214:483–7.

43. Bayne KA, Dexter SL, Strange GM. The effects of food treat provisioning and human interaction on the behavioral well-being of rhesus monkeys. Contemp Top Lab Anim Sci 1993;32:6–9.

A Framework for Solving Behavior Problems

Parvene Farhoody, MA

KEYWORDS

- Behavior • Behavior analysis • Applied behavior analysis • Functional assessment

KEY POINTS

- Solving behavior problems begins with a basic understanding of the principles of learning.
- Applied behavior analysis approaches solutions to real-world behavior problems with the same commitment to objective analysis and systematic data collection that characterizes experimental behavior analysis.
- The building blocks of learning involve 4 basic elements: positive and negative reinforcement and positive and negative punishment.

INTRODUCTION

Solving behavior problems begins with a basic understanding of the principles of learning. However, to change behavior effectively and efficiently, it is necessary to examine the function that the problem behavior serves for the animal. Applied behavior analysis (ABA) quantifies and measures observable behavior in applied settings and uses direct and indirect functional assessments to identify the function of behavior. Advances in the treatment of problem behavior using ABA have predominantly been made through work with humans with special needs. These same advances have been applied to nonhuman species with equally compelling effects. Functional behavioral assessments (FBAs) are the tools used to develop and test hypotheses about the environmental factors' controlling behavior, in other words, the purpose or function that the behavior serves for the individual. Functional assessment is the first step in implementing a systematic behavior-change strategy. Behavior analysis is a data-driven science; therefore, treatment is always based on empirical data, and all changes made to a behavioral intervention are based on these data. Behavior change strategies include antecedent interventions and training alternative behaviors that serve the same function as the problem behavior. ABA continues to advance as a science through the exchange of information between practitioners and through the process of peer-reviewed publication.

The author has nothing to disclose.
Department of Psychology, Queens College, Graduate Center of the City University of New York, 65-30 Kissena Boulevard, Flushing, NY 11367, USA
E-mail addresses: parvene@behaviormatters.com; pfarhoody@gc.cuny.edu

In 1968, 3 influential figures in behavior analysis described the defining features of behavior analysis. Twenty years later, these same behavior analysts noted that these dimensions were still current. The defining characteristics that signify the work called ABA are as follows: applied, behavioral, analytic, technological, conceptually systematic, effective, and capable of generalized outcomes.[1,2]

ABA approaches solutions to real-world behavior problems with the same commitment to objective analysis and systematic data collection that characterizes experimental behavior analysis. The goal of systematic manipulation is to demonstrate a cause-and-effect relationship between an independent variable (the intervention/ treatment protocol implemented to change a behavior) and the dependent variable (the behavior targeted for change/new behavior produced).[3] (See the article by Farhoody elsewhere in this issue titled, Behavior Analysis: The Science of Training.) As with all science, the assumptions of behavior analysis are deterministic; all behavior has causes and serves a function for the organism, and these functional relationships between the environment and the organism control behavior. Therefore, to approach a behavior problem systematically, it is necessary (1) to have a working hypothesis about which environmental stimuli are maintaining a problem behavior and then (2) to alter or eliminate those environmental variables, thereby altering or eliminating the problem behavior. As with all procedures designed to show experimental control, demonstrating causal relationships can be challenging. This is especially true in applied settings, where it can be difficult to ensure any environmental control. Solving the behavior problem is paramount; however, collecting objective data is essential to verify that the intervention procedure did in fact cause the behavior change. Without this, there may indeed have been successful behavior change, but successful change without the analysis of behavior leaves the teacher with little ability to predict and control behavior. Perhaps most importantly, an understanding of the behavioral mechanisms responsible for success is essential for replication by other practitioners. When results can be replicated, they can be improved so that each subsequent intervention procedure becomes more effective and efficient than the previous one. The ultimate goal for using the behavior analytic systematic approach is to advance a behavioral technology and eliminate hit-or-miss procedures. Behavior analysis advances as a science, and as a technology, when systematic treatment procedures implemented by ABA practitioners are shared, examined, discussed, and refined by contributions from other colleagues. It cannot be overemphasized that the data-driven, peer-review processes of behavior analysis are defining features of the applied science.

BEHAVIORAL MECHANISMS

The building blocks of learning involve 4 basic elements: positive and negative reinforcement and positive and negative punishment. The almost infinite numbers of possibilities arising from these building blocks are the tools of the behavioral technician. If that seems like an exaggeration, consider that only 4 nucleotide bases make up DNA. The combination of these 4 make up millions of life forms. Although a working understanding of these basic learning mechanisms is mandatory for dissecting behavior if the goal is to become fluent at solving behavior problems; even a cursory examination of these basics can provide insight about why behavior occurs and how it can be changed. Because behavior happens and changes around us every day, it is easy to underestimate its complexity. Most behavior occurs without awareness: brushing your teeth, driving to work, physically moving, thinking, and exercising self-control, along with complex clusters of behaviors such as raising a child. These are all made up of countless permutations of behavior changes. However, when a particular behavior is in need of change, attention is drawn to it, and when this happens, it is often goes unrealized that behavior is a natural science, and like all natural phenomena, it obeys laws. Behavior analysis takes the view that behavior is a physical phenomenon and that it can be controlled. The idea that behavior analysis is a powerful tool to control behavior has been a large contributor to the public's often-apprehensive view of it. Effective tools can be can be used for nefarious means. A sharp knife is a very effective tool that will cut well if used properly, and therefore it needs to be used carefully. Behavior analysis is a very effective tool to change behavior, and it too should be used with care. The potential for misuse should no more lead us to dispense with sharp knives as tools than to dismiss an effective behavioral change technology. (For an interesting discussion on the criticism of behavior analysis and the ethics of behavior change, see Chance.[4])

BEHAVIOR IS QUANTIFIABLE

A typical human being in the 21st century who breathes, sees, walks, eats, and eliminates does not tend to think much about these processes. However, if he gets sick, he generally turns to a trained professional for systematic diagnoses and treatment. In behavior analysis as in medicine, a diagnosis is based on empirical evidence. To say that a dog bites because it is dominant is the behavioral equivalent of proclaiming that a patient has a fever because the hot spirit possesses him. Hypothetical constructs, which are simply variables that cannot be measured or verified, such as *mean*, *stubborn*, and *spoiled*, or *intelligent* and *sweet*, are not the realm of behavior analysis. Behavior analysts measure observable behavior using operational definitions. Operationalized behavior is behavior that has been described in such painstaking detail that anyone could recognize when it was or was not occurring. When behavior is described as methodically as would be any other scientific dependent or independent variable, then change to behavior can be objectively determined.

When making a diagnosis of a behavior problem, the first measurement of the target behavior is made in a baseline condition, before any intervention has been implemented. Measurement continues throughout the intervention and after the treatment has been withdrawn or a maintenance plan has been put into place. During this process, changes are made on the basis of data and are not arbitrary. Whether a treatment is considered successful is based on the data returned, which indicate changes in the dimension(s) of the behavior being measured (ie, increases or decreases in frequency, duration, magnitude, latency, etc). This process is familiar to every trained scientist. For example, in medicine, when a patient presents with a fever, established diagnostics are implemented to determine the cause. Empirical data from a blood sample, for example, show elevated white blood cells, and a hypothesis is made on the basis of the practitioner's biologic education, which informs him or her that an increase in white blood cells is often the result of infection; therefore, an antibiotic is prescribed. The fever is a symptom that was measured, the cause is a presumed infection, and a treatment is implemented. Whether the medical practitioner's assumption is correct cannot be known until the results of treatment are measured. After treatment, data are again collected, and the next course of action is based on the data. It is critical to understand the systematic approach of ABA if one is to distinguish it from other behavior modification approaches. It is not so much that behavior cannot be changed any other way; it is that the use of behavioral technology has been shown to save time and to avoid behavior change techniques that might worsen the problem.[5,6] Behavior analysis allows behavior science to advance and improve with each generation, as opposed to information being passed down anecdotally.

LEARNING THE ABCs

Behavior is a cross-species phenomenon; regardless of the organism whose behavior is targeted for change, the mechanisms and the processes for learning and behavior change remain the same. At this time, the vast majority of applied behavioral research is done with humans. The research amassed from advances in the field of ABA over the last 60 years has expanded our understanding of learning processes and the principles and laws that govern behavior. (See *The Journal of Applied Behavior Analysis* or *The Journal of the Experimental Analysis of Behavior* for published research.) Today's behavior analyst thinks far outside the Skinner box. The following are a few examples of derived principles in the science of behavior that are, in and of themselves, entire fields of study (for a more detailed look at some of these behavioral phenomena, see Mazur[7]):

- Behavioral economics informs our understanding of the factors responsible for the allocation of energy to one behavior over another.
- Behavioral momentum theory provides mathematical precision to predicting a behavior's resistance to change.
- The increasingly deeper understanding of schedules of reinforcement, properties of discriminative stimuli, and conditioned reinforcers have demonstrated that throughout the continuum of complexity in the relationship between organism and environment, behavior continues to act lawfully.

Table 1 outlines the 4 basic learning mechanisms underlying all behavior change. It is not uncommon for the 4 learning processes to become confused when trying to identify them within the context of physical activity. To use these effectively, it is useful to remember the following 3 constants to help keep the learning mechanism distinctly different:

- Always define the behavior of interest *first.*
- *Positive* means addition; *negative* means subtraction.
- *Reinforcement* means increase; *punishment* means decrease.

CHANGING BEHAVIOR

The first step for the behavior analyst when confronted with a behavior problem is to operationalize the behavior targeted for change in as much detail as possible. The easier it is to identify the target behavior (the dependent variable), the more precisely a change can be made. After the target behavior has been clearly defined, measurement of a behavioral dimension is taken under baseline conditions. The behavioral dimension(s) chosen for measurement provides quantitative information about changes that

Table 1 Basic learning mechanisms			
Operation	Change in Response Strength	Terminology	Alternate Terminology
Stimulus presented	Increase	Positive reinforcement	
Stimulus removed	Increase	Negative reinforcement	Escape or avoidance
Stimulus presented	Decrease	Positive punishment	Type 1 punishment
Stimulus removed	Decrease	Negative punishment	Type 2 punishment or response cost

occurred during the intervention. Some measurements that may be useful are the frequency, magnitude, and duration of the behavior or the latency between responses. (For a comprehensive look at measuring behavior, see Martin and Bateson.[8])

The following is an example of an operationalized definition of a behavior originally described by the animal's caretaker as "The dog is always begging for food."

"Begging Behavior":

- The dog's body is in any position within a 4-ft radius of a person eating food. The dog may engage in any of the following behaviors: looking directly at the person eating, being silent, whining, barking, or touching the person eating with any part of its body.
- It is considered begging behavior if the dog is outside a 4-ft radius of the person eating food and is engaging in any sort of vocalization: whining, barking, growling, and so forth.
- It is not considered begging behavior if the dog is outside a 4-ft radius and is only engaged in looking at the person eating food.

The process of operationalizing a behavior may seem tedious, but this degree of specificity makes it possible for all those interacting with the animal to recognize when and when not to reinforce behavior. An operational definition can also be changed or amended if needed, allowing for more precise training. This description, along with the data collected during this particular intervention procedure, will make the next application of the intervention more efficient.

REINFORCEMENT MAINTAINS BEHAVIOR

Reinforcement is a basic learning phenomenon; it is a *procedure defined by its effect*. Reinforcement maintains or increases the frequency of a behavior when it is contingent on that behavior. Reinforcement is a behavioral principle and it is lawful. The statement, "I reinforced the behavior and it stopped" is not much different from the statement, "I threw an apple into the air and it did not fall." Reinforcement occurs as defined: it maintains or increases the frequency of behavior on which it is contingent. If a behavior stops occurring, it could not have been reinforced. Punishment decreases behavior. Punishment can be defined by its effect. The statement, "I punished my parrot for screaming and he screamed more" is as meaningless as the previous statement. These 2 examples simply illustrate how confusing behavioral terminology can become when it is used casually. No one would say, "The cat was anesthetized and was wide awake." This is immediately recognized as senseless; if the cat is wide-awake, it is not anesthetized. If the cat had gone through a process of being anesthetized and was wide-awake, then the anesthetizing process must have been incorrectly applied. The incorrect application of anesthesia resulted in the cat's remaining awake. This makes sense to any trained veterinarian. For the behavior analyst, the mechanisms of behavior and the terminology used to describe those mechanisms require the same level of specificity that one would find in any field of science. The difference with behavioral science, however, is that few scientific specialties have terminology that is also used in the common vernacular, so the incorrect use of behavioral terminology can be a source of confusion.

FUNCTIONAL RELATIONSHIPS

Because there is a cause-and-effect relationship between the occurrence of behavior and the environment, it follows that if the relationship between the target behavior and specific environmental factors can be determined, then those environmental factors can be altered and the behavior changed. Skinner's 3-term contingency is the "formula" used to analyze behavior and discover the functional relationships between events. When a behavior is dependent, or contingent, on a specific event(s) in the environment, it is functional; it "works." If you change the environment, you change the behavior: if x happens, then y happens. All behavior can be divided into 3 terms $(S^D:R_1 \rightarrow S^R)$[9] or the simplified version $(A:B \rightarrow C)$.[3] A discriminative stimulus/antecedent (S^D or A) sets the occasion for a behavior (R_1 or B) to occur, and the consequence (S^R or C) follows only if the behavior occurred. This is the basis for all analysis of the relationship between the environment (A and C) and the organism (B).

The relationship between an antecedent, a behavior, and a consequence is said to be functional when the following 3 conditions are met:

- The behavior is operationally defined and performed by the animal whose behavior we are trying to change.
- The consequence is a description of an environmental event, and the appearance of the consequence depends on the behavior occurring first.
- The antecedent is a description of an environmental event, and the behavior it precedes depends on the antecedent to occur.

FUNCTIONS OF BEHAVIOR

In 1977, Carr[10] examined possible motivations for self-injurious behavior in human beings. In 1982, Iwata and colleagues[6] used functional analysis (FA) to experimentally examine motivation and the behavioral mechanisms that might maintain this undesired behavior in developmentally disabled participants. In other words, Iwata and colleagues[6] used FA as a diagnostic tool to identify the functional relationship between self-injurious behavior and the environment; what purpose did this behavior serve for these individuals? FA refers to the manipulation of environmental events under controlled conditions to determine the functions of behavior. Behavior analysts working with animals also use FA as a diagnostic tool to examine possible functions of problem behavior in nonhuman species. **Fig. 1** shows the behavioral mechanisms identified as possible reinforcers for problem behavior by Iwata and colleagues.[6]

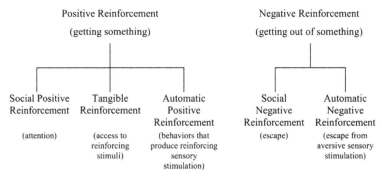

Functions of Behavior

Fig. 1. Functions of behavior.

FUNCTIONAL BEHAVIORAL ASSESSMENTS

The tools used by behavior analysts to determine functional relationships between behavior and the environment are called FBAs. FBAs are a way to develop and test hypotheses about the environmental factors' controlling behavior (ie, the purpose or function the behavior serves for the individual). The same behavioral topography can serve different functions, so what the animal does, in and of itself, does not tell the entire behavioral story. For example, a child may spill her glass of milk at each meal for many reasons: to get attention, to escape eating a particular food, to get sympathy from one or both parents or a sibling. The milk-spilling behavior may be the behavior targeted for change, and it may have the same topography each time it occurs; however, finding the most effective and efficient approach to solving the behavior will be found by addressing the function of the behavior.

FBAs can take many forms. Indirect assessment includes several standardized evaluation tools, questionnaires, and checklists that have been created to help caretakers of humans with special needs provide information that can assist in leading the behavior analyst to form hypotheses. Indirect assessments gather background information that may be helpful in identifying factors that influence problem behavior; however, indirect assessments are limited in the sense that they rely on subjective information. When using indirect assessments, it is important to pose questions that lead to answers that are descriptions of behavior rather than constructs or explanatory fictions. Constructs and explanatory fictions can be thought of as labels that describe what an animal "is" rather than descriptions of what an animal "does." For example, "the monkey is stubborn" rather than "the monkey moves away from the door when asked to exit the enclosure." (For more about the problem with constructs, see the article by Farhoody elsewhere in this issue titled, *Behavior Analysis: The Science of Training*.) Indirect assessments provide valuable information, but direct assessment of behavior is the most desirable method of data collection.

FUNCTIONAL ANALYSIS

FA, also called experimental analysis, is the most controlled direct assessment procedure. Results of these assessments are considered confirmation of function rather than hypotheses. Although conducting a full FA can be time-consuming, FA has been shown to identify reinforcing events with a high percentage of accuracy.[3,5,6,11] By using this highly controlled procedure to identify what is maintaining problem behavior, it is less likely that time will be wasted on interventions that may not be successful or that the intervention will increase the problem behavior.[6] The following is a skeletal description of the diagnostic procedure:

- Identify and operationalize the target behavior.
- Systematically arrange several reinforcing scenarios to simulate different reinforcement contingencies.
- Present each contingency independently, and measure the effect on behavior of each condition.

For example, it is hypothesized that for a particular chimpanzee, throwing feces is maintained by social positive reinforcement. Several conditions are tested to dispute or verify this hypothesis. A controlled setting is purposefully arranged so the primate will engage in the problem behavior (throwing feces), and the immediate consequence will be that a preferred human appears and talks to the primate. The social reinforcement hypothesis is tested along with 2 or 3 other hypotheses. Possible scenarios might include the following: throwing feces is maintained by negative social reinforcement (escape). The primate is asked to perform a task, and when the primate engages in the problem behavior, the task request is removed; throwing feces is maintained by tangible reinforcement. The chimpanzee throws feces and a keeper gives him a preferred object to keep him occupied. These testing situations are done in several predescribed trials with the goal of measuring the effect of the different consequences on the problem behavior. If the feces-throwing behavior increased with each occurrence of the social positive reinforcement test condition, this would support the initial hypothesis that positive social reinforcement was in fact the reinforcer maintaining the behavior, and an intervention would be designed to accommodate this function. However, if the behavior decreased in the social positive reinforcement condition and increased in the negative social reinforcement condition, an intervention would be designed to accommodate a different function.

FA can be very useful; however, this sort of direct manipulation is often difficult if not impossible to conduct in applied settings. This is especially true when there is limited time, funding, and/or staff or if there is the risk that even brief occurrences of additional reinforcement might temporarily increase the behavior problem or involve risk. Another limitation of FA is the ability to set up situations in contrived settings that are similar enough to reality to elicit the problem behavior. Because FA allows conclusions to be drawn about the variables maintaining behavior before putting any behavioral intervention into place, it is the standard to which other FBAs are held, and it is desirable to conduct a full FA whenever possible. Kahng and Iwata[12] studied 2 abbreviated methods of conducting FA and found them to be almost 70% as accurate as the more extensive procedure. These quick yet accurate procedures provide even more incentive to use FA before treatment.

DESCRIPTIVE FUNCTIONAL ASSESSMENT

Descriptive FBAs are also tools for determining the function of a problem behavior. The difference between an FA and a functional assessment is that in the latter, the subject is observed in its natural environment and engaged in its typical routine. Descriptive functional assessment is most useful when the assessment describes the specific environmental events that precede (antecedent) and follow (consequence) occurrences of the problem behavior. Continuous recording or time sampling can be conducted on behavior in real time or can be collected using video recordings and then scored later.[8] These data provide structured information about the antecedents and consequences surrounding the problem behavior. A sample ABC narrative recording chart is shown in **Fig. 2**. Other diagnostic tools, such as scatter plot analysis of the time, place, and people/animals that might have been present when the problem behavior occurred, can also help discover patterns of environmental events that are correlated with the problem behavior. Through these procedures, hypotheses can be made about the more probable functions of the problem behavior and less probable functions are ruled out.

TESTING THE HYPOTHESIS

After conducting an FBA, the practitioner is in a better position to plan and implement treatment. Although it is certainly possible to implement an intervention without conducting a systematic functional assessment, it has been demonstrated with human subjects that interventions based on an FBA are more likely to be effective than arbitrarily chosen interventions.[5,6,11] Three main strategic interventions are used to alter the relationship between the antecedent, behavior, and consequence so as to alter

ABC Narrative Recording Form

Individual observed _____   Date _____

Observer _____

Time begin _____ AM PM   Time end _____ AM PM

Antecedent (explain the events that come before the behavior)	Behavior (explain exactly what the animal did—the actual behavior)	Consequence (explain the events that followed the behavior or occurred as a result of the behavior)

Fig. 2. ABC narrative recording form. (*Data from* Cooper JO, Heron TE, Heward WL. Applied behavior analysis. 2nd edition. Upper Saddle River (NJ): Pearson Education; 2007.)

the occurrence of the problem behavior. The 3 strategic approaches are altering the antecedents, altering the consequences, and teaching alternative behaviors.

Altering the Antecedent

One of the most effective and underused approaches to solving behavior problems is altering antecedent stimuli. As discussed in *Behavior Analysis: The Science Behind the Training,* in the operant conditioning paradigm, antecedents do not cause behavior; they only set the occasion for the behavior to occur. There are 2 ways to alter antecedent stimuli:

1. *Change the antecedent stimuli that signal the opportunity for reinforcement.* It is established that the behavior is maintained by reinforcement, so removing the

stimulus that signals the opportunity to acquire reinforcement will make the behavior less likely to occur. Often this surprisingly simple intervention requires nothing more than a small manipulation of the environment. *Example:* A child with autism has difficulty using a bar of soap in the tub, preferring to constantly drop the soap and watch it hit the water than to rub it on his body. The antecedent intervention is to replace the bar of soap with liquid soap and a washcloth.

2. *Alter the motivating operation that gives the consequence its value.* Motivating operations are unconditioned or conditioned antecedent stimuli that increase or decrease the value of a reinforcer or any behavior that has led to that reinforcer in the past. A very simplistic example would be the following: thirst is a motivating operation that increases the value of water as a reinforcer and increases the behavior of drinking out of a water fountain, because that behavior has led to water in the past. This fourth variable is placed before the ABC and provides information about the probability that a behavior will occur. For more on motivating operations, see Michael.[13] *Example:* A narcotics detection dog is given access to a highly preferred toy only when engaged in detection work. Deprivation of the preferred toy increases the motivating operation of play, thereby increasing the value of the preferred toy as reinforcer and increasing the frequency of all behaviors that led to that reinforcer in the past (ie, finding narcotics).

Altering the Consequence

This is usually the most common strategy employed when approaching behavior problems. The simplest change to decrease a problem behavior is to stop providing all reinforcement to that behavior. When a behavior that was reinforced in the past is no longer reinforced, that behavior is "put on extinction." This procedure alone is often sufficient to decrease the frequency of a problem behavior to a degree that makes it no longer a problem. However, extinction is most often implemented as part of a differential reinforcement procedure (see *Teaching Alternative Behaviors*), so that some other desired behavior is given reinforcement instead of the problem behavior. Another alternative consequence change used to decrease behavior is to add a punisher after an occurrence of the problem behavior in place of the reinforcing consequence; however, this may result in other, undesirable behaviors, such as aggressive behavior or fear responses. Therefore, to avoid this risk, it is advantageous whenever possible, to choose extinction or a combination of extinction with the next strategy, teaching alternative behaviors. *Example:* A horse has a history of getting carrots (tangible reinforcement) after it pushes its nose at the pocket/body of the owner. The owner no longer gives carrots if the horse is pushing on her pocket/body.

Teaching Alternative Behaviors

The goal of this strategy is to *teach a replacement behavior that is the functional equivalent of the problem behavior.* After a new behavior is trained, the problem behavior can be put on extinction; all reinforcement is removed for any occurrence of the problem behavior, and the new alternative behavior receives all the reinforcement previously allocated to the problem behavior. This sort of replacement allows the animal to engage in an alternative behavior that results in the same consequence as the problem behavior. The animal continues to get reinforced at the same rate, but the behavior being reinforced has changed. Reinforcement increases the frequency of the behavior it is contingent upon, so to increase the probability of success of the intervention, it is desirable to provide the alternative behavior with even more reinforcement than was originally provided to the problem behavior. The baseline data collected before the intervention will provide information about the amount of reinforcement previously given to the problem behavior and will indicate how much reinforcement to give the alternative behavior. If the hypothesis about the function of the problem behavior was correct, after the problem behavior is put on extinction and reinforcement is given to the functionally equivalent replacement behavior, a decrease in occurrence of problem behavior will be observed. Example: Building on the extinction example above, the horse is taught to put its nose on a target stick for carrots (tangible reinforcement). After this, the behavior of the horse pushing its nose on the pocket/body of the owner is put on extinction. Undesirable behavior is extinguished, and the horse is now reinforced for engaging in the new desired behavior. A decrease in problem behavior is less likely if the new behavior does not serve the same function as the problem behavior. If touching the target stick resulted in rubs (positive social reinforcement) instead of carrots (tangible reinforcement), the problem behavior might not decrease in frequency at all, or might continue at a higher rate than it would if the consequence continued to be a tangible reinforcer.[3,5,11]

DIFFERENTIAL REINFORCEMENT

Differential reinforcement is a procedure in which 2 or more behaviors are reinforced at different rates. For example, differential reinforcement schedules are often used in combination with extinction. One behavior is given no reinforcement to decrease its frequency while other behavior(s) receives a high rate of reinforcement to increase its frequency. The behavior chosen for reinforcement is determined from the information gathered in the FBA. The most desirable replacement behavior is one that serves the same function as the problem behavior. Three commonly used differential reinforcement schedules are:

- DRO—Differential reinforcement of other behavior: the animal is reinforced for engaging in any behavior other than the problem behavior.
- DRA—Differential reinforcement of an alternative behavior: the animal is reinforced for performing a particular alternative behavior. (This behavior could be one already in the animal's repertoire or one specifically taught.)
- DRI—Differential reinforcement of incompatible behavior: the animal is reinforced for engaging in a behavior that it cannot perform at the same time it is engaged in the problem behavior. (This behavior could be one already in the animal's repertoire or one specifically taught.)

Examples: Returning to the feces-throwing chimpanzee, observation and measurement of the behavior in baseline and a descriptive functional assessment led to the hypothesis that throwing feces is being maintained by positive social reinforcement. The data collected at baseline are now used to decide when and how the intervention will be implemented. Information might include when the chimpanzee was most likely to have engaged in the problem behavior and who were the preferred handlers. An observation schedule is put into place so the chimpanzee can be reinforced whenever it engages in desired behavior. At those moments, the handler will appear to talk and play with the chimpanzee. The function of throwing feces was to get positive social reinforcement from the preferred handler. The intervention teaches the animal that this same reinforcer is now available for engaging in a different behavior. If the intervention were a DRO, the chimpanzee might be reinforced when engaged in *anything* other than feces-throwing. A DRA intervention might be to train the animal to engage in play with a specific toy and, when the animal is engaged in play, reinforcement occurs. In a DRI, the animal might be taught to hold a particular object with both hands for reinforcement. This incompatible behavior would make it impossible to pick up and throw feces while holding the object. All these differential reinforcement schedules result in an increase in the desired behavior and a decrease in feces throwing.

The purpose of data collection is to increase the likelihood of intervention success and to make clear how the intervention was responsible for the change. Through this process, it is possible to develop a catalog of effective behavior-changing protocols that provide specific information that allows all those working with a particular animal to be extremely consistent and give the animal every opportunity to continually improve. Operationally defined behaviors and a detailed protocol for the behavior of the human caregivers allow for efficient and effective behavior change and the production of strong, persistent, desirable behavior.[14] For examples of the use of behavior analytic interventions conducted with differential reinforcement, see Dorey and colleagues,[15] Martin and colleagues,[16] Ferguson and Rosales-Ruiz,[17] and Slater and Dymond.[18]

MAINTENANCE

The final and very important part of any behavioral intervention is a plan for how the behavior change will be maintained. This area is often overlooked, which leads to a return of the problem behavior even after initial success in producing change. In some ways, a good maintenance plan requires the greatest understanding of behavioral science. Many factors are involved in why behavioral responses do or do not persist: how the behavior was acquired, the behavior's history of reinforcement, response strength, motivating operations, stimulus and response generalization, the value of the reinforcer, and still yet other factors. For a maintenance plan to be successful, the function of the behavior must be kept foremost in mind, and both the function of behavior and the value of the reinforcers must be reassessed on a regular basis. The broader the understanding of behavior science, the more a training plan can be a clear road map on how to get from here to there. ABA offers ways to improve our lives and the lives of others. As with practitioners of any science, the more comprehensive the knowledge of the practitioner, the more he or she can contribute to the advancement of the science.

REFERENCES

1. Baer DM, Wolf MM, Risley TR. Some current dimensions of applied behavior analysis. J Exp Anal Behav 1968;1:91–7.
2. Baer DM, Wolf MM, Risley TR. Some still-current dimensions of applied behavior analysis. J Appl Behav Anal 1987;20:313–27.
3. Cooper JO, Heron TE, Heward WL. Applied behavior analysis. 2nd edition. Upper Saddle River (NJ): Pearson Education; 2007.
4. Chance P. First course in applied behavior analysis. Pacific Grove (CA): Brooks/ Cole; 1998.
5. Day RM, Rea JA, Schussler NG, et al. A functionally based approach to the treatment of self-injurious behavior. Behav Modif 1988;12:565–89.
6. Iwata B, Dorsey M, Slifer K, et al. Toward a functional analysis of self-injury. Anal Interv Dev Disabil 1982;2:3–20 (Reprinted in J Appl Behav Anal 1994;27: 196–209).
7. Mazur JE. Learning and behavior. 6th edition. Upper Saddle River (NJ): Pearson; 2006.
8. Martin P, Bateson P. Measuring behaviour: an introductory guide. 2nd edition. Cambridge (UK): Cambridge University Press; 1993.

9. Skinner BF. The behavior of organisms. New York: Appleton-Century-Crofts; 1938.
10. Carr EG. The motivation of self-injurious behavior: a review of some hypotheses. Psychol Bull 1977;84:800–16.
11. Iwata BA, Pace GM, Dorsey MF, et al. The functions of self-injurious behavior: an experimental-epidemiological analysis. J Appl Behav Anal 1994;27:215–40.
12. Kahng SW, Iwata BA. Correspondence between outcomes of brief and extended functional analyses. J Appl Behav Anal 1999;32:149–59.
13. Michael J. Distinguishing between discriminative and motivational functions of stimuli. J Exp Anal Behav 1982;37:149–55.
14. Horner RH. Functional assessment: contributions and future directions. J Appl Behav Anal 1994;27:401–4.
15. Dorey NR, Rosales-Ruiz J, Smith R, et al. Functional analysis and treatment of self-injury in a captive olive baboon. J Appl Behav Anal 2009;42:785–94.
16. Martin AL, Bloomsmith MA, Kelley ME, et al. Functional analysis and treatment of human-directed undesirable behavior exhibited by a captive chimpanzee. J Appl Behav Anal 2011;44:139–43.
17. Ferguson DL, Rosales-Ruiz J. Loading the problem loader: the effects of target training and shaping on trailer-loading behavior of horses. J Appl Behav Anal 2001;34:409–24.
18. Slater C, Dymond S. Using differential reinforcement to improve equine welfare: shaping appropriate truck loading and feet handling. Behav Processes 2011; 86:329–39.

Marine Mammal Training
The History of Training Animals for Medical Behaviors and Keys to Their Success

Ken Ramirez

KEYWORDS

• Marine mammals • Training • Husbandry training • Medical training

KEY POINTS

- Training is an important key to improving animal care, and the use of positive reinforcement is essential to successful medical behavior training.
- There are many foundational behaviors that an animal must learn to be able to successfully learn and maintain medical behaviors.
- The training of some medical behaviors takes time; they cannot be rushed or the benefits of training will be lost.
- Medical behaviors must be practiced frequently to maintain their usefulness.
- Use the information learned from previous training of individual behaviors to aid in successful training with new animals and new species.

INTRODUCTION

The training of both domestic and exotic species for participation in medical behaviors is a helpful tool in the care and management of individual animals. The practice of training individual animals to help in their own health care is difficult to trace back to its origins. The use of these techniques on large exotic mammals became commonplace only as recently as the late 1990s and early 2000s. However, the practice seems to have been perfected and made popular with marine mammal species, starting in the 1970s. The development of better training techniques for a variety of medical behaviors is a foundational key worth examining and has been proved to be applicable across species.

OPERANT CONDITIONING

Marine mammals, particularly cetaceans (dolphins and whales), first began being trained using operant conditioning in the 1940s at Marine Studios of Florida scientific techniques were introduced by Keller Breland of Animal Behavior Enterprises. Dolphins were poorly understood at that time and seldom seen by the public. The

The author has nothing to disclose.
Shedd Aquarium, 1200 South Lake Shore Drive, Chicago, IL 60605, USA
E-mail address: kramirez@sheddaquarium.org

Vet Clin Exot Anim 15 (2012) 413–423
http://dx.doi.org/10.1016/j.cvex.2012.06.005   **vetexotic.theclinics.com**

attraction was first built as a studio to allow movie and television productions a place to create underwater movie sets. The trainability of the dolphins was noted and the facility became a popular tourist attraction.[1] This led to additional exploration of the learning abilities of the dolphins and expanded on the use of operant conditioning throughout the marine mammal community, which eventually led to the training of a wide variety of medical behaviors.

POSITIVE REINFORCEMENT

Pinnipeds (seals and sea lions) were involved in training programs that predated dolphins by several decades; although positive reinforcement was used to some extent with seals and sea lions, some traditional punishment techniques were also used in the training of some sea lions. The key to successful training and maintenance of medical behaviors was a focus on the use of positive reinforcement techniques. This approach minimized or eliminated the use of coercion and punishment to gain the animal's cooperation and created a trusting relationship between the keeper or trainer and the animal. This was first demonstrated in the work of Karen Pryor at Sea Life Park in Hawaii in the 1960s.[2,3] As these relationships grew; the types of medical behaviors that could be trained also grew.

MANAGEMENT BEHAVIORS

Prior to starting to train more complex medical behaviors, marine mammal trainers established several key basic behaviors with each animal. Success at training difficult medical behaviors necessitated several key foundational behaviors in each animal's repertoire; often these behaviors were referred to as management behaviors. Without a solid foundation of trained management behaviors, it was discovered that medical behaviors were far more difficult to train and maintain. These behaviors included, but were not limited to:

- Eating from the hand: This brought the animals close enough to be worked with and trained more effectively.
- Stationing: This taught animals a position to come to for each training session, usually close to and in front of the trainer.
- Gating: It was important that animals be able to be moved as a group and as individuals from one enclosure to another. Animals needed to be comfortable being separated through a gate or doorway from the rest of their group.
- Tactile: As trust developed, animals learned to allow the trainers to touch them, which would ultimately assist with many medical behaviors.
- Targeting: Most animals were taught to touch some part of their body to another object, referred to as a target. The procedure of targeting is a useful tool in guiding animals into proper position for medical training.[4,5]

SHOW TRAINING

Marine mammal training became best known due to the wide exposure in shows at zoos, aquariums, and marine parks throughout the world. The techniques used for shows later became useful in the development of methods to train medical behaviors. This is evident in reviewing the growth and development of training through the professional organization of marine mammal trainers, the International Marine Animal Trainers Association (IMATA), which was first formed in the early 1970s. A review of the publications from IMATA indicates a shift in focus from show behaviors to medical behaviors began in the late 1970s.[6]

DESENSITIZATION

Trainers had to rely on the science of behavior analysis and develop a better understanding of various learning theories to successfully train medical behaviors. Desensitization techniques became key tools in preparing animals for exposure to needles, new smells, the presence of veterinarians, and other unique stimuli that might be associated with various medical behaviors. The most important of these concepts were:

- Habituation: The exposure to new stimuli repeatedly over time such that the animal gradually becomes accustomed to the stimuli and accepts it.
- Counterconditioning: Controlled exposure to a new stimuli, paired with positive reinforcement, to essentially train the animal to get accustomed to the new stimuli and gradually transition it from a scary or uncomfortable experience for the animal into one that is accepted and in some cases enjoyed.[7]

KEY BEHAVIORS

The marine mammal community realized an exponential growth in the spread of several key medical behaviors and the development of improved techniques through the sharing of information facilitated by their professional organization, IMATA. As demonstrated in the many examples below, discussions about possibilities of training medical behaviors began taking place in the late 1970s[8]; the first examples of success were reported on in the early 1980s, and by the late 1980s the training of medical behaviors became commonplace. Following are a few of the most common medical behaviors trained and some of the key aspects shared and learned over the years of training those behaviors.

VENIPUNCTURE (TAKING BLOOD)

Because of the wealth of important data gained from blood sampling, this behavior became the biggest goal for most marine mammal facilities as they began exploring medical training. In 1984 the first two formal reports were published describing the successful techniques used to train blood taking with killer whales at Sea World in San Diego[9] and Hawaiian monk seals at the Waikiki Aquarium in Honolulu.[10] By 1990, formal reports and presentations reported on the training of blood taking in bottlenose dolphins,[11–15] California sea lions,[11,12,14,16–18] walruses,[12,14,16] and penguins.[11,12,14] As the number of species and facilities grew that had achieved success, the key elements to those successes were widely documented and have since proven to be successful with a wide variety of species, not just marine mammals. A few of these key elements have included:

- Gradual desensitization: Because of the potential discomfort for the animal in having a needle inserted, the process of getting animal used to the process should not be rushed and the foundational behaviors leading up to needle insertion need to be well established (calm animal, length of time staying still gradually increased, number of people present gradually increased, etc).[4,7,9,13]
- Practice the procedure without the discomfort of actual needle insertion far more often than doing an actual blood draw. Some resources suggest a minimum of at least 100 practices for each single actual procedure.[4,5,14–16]
- Teach the animal to accept variety: Because the sensation of a needle insertion cannot be accurately recreated at every training session, when practicing the procedure of touching the animal, change the sensation by regularly varying how and with what the animal is touched (terry cloth towel, a trainer's knuckles,

a sharp object, spray of water, etc). This teaches the animal not to expect any one type of tactile sensation and often assists them in being more accepting of the unique sensation of a needle insertion.[5]

SEPARATION, REMOVAL, KENNELING

In the medical care of almost any species, there becomes a need to separate an animal from the group, move it into a kennel, stretcher, or cage, and to move or transport it. Although this had been done since the beginning of zoological animal care, the systematic training of these things using behavioral control and carefully planned desensitization steps was well documented in the marine mammal community in the 1980s.[16,18–21] The lessons learned from each of these early examples have been used in the training of many similar behaviors with a wide variety of species in subsequent years, a few of those key concepts include the following:

- Gradual desensitization and practicing often apply to this behavior and most other medical behaviors as described previously in the section on blood taking.
- Do not trap the animal: In the early stages of training, do not trap the animal; give the animal the option to back away or get out. This increases their likeliness to participate and that separation or moving is not going to result in fear-inducing circumstances
- Make it a positive experience: Because separation, kenneling, and removal frequently are associated with discomfort or aversive experiences, it is essential that the animal have many brief and positive experiences after complying with the requested behavior; limiting uncomfortable experiences to very rare occurrences.

STOMACH TUBE

The insertion of a tube down the throat of an animal is not as commonly used with terrestrial animals, and the lack of a gag reflex probably makes this an easier behavior to train with dolphins and whales than most other species. For that reason, the insertion of a stomach tube became a fairly commonly trained behavior with dolphins and whales.[12,14,22,23] However, as the techniques for stomach tube insertion were being perfected, several facilities began having success training the behavior in pinnipeds.[24] The development of the stomach tube behavior proved useful in accomplishing other goals besides simple hydration of the animal:

- Administration of medication or fluids: In addition to allowing trainers to hydrate or give fluids and food to an animal, the use of the stomach tube proved useful in the administration of vitamins or medications when needed.
- Sampling gastric contents: Veterinarians were able to use the behavior to get gastric samples from the animals. Gastric contents could be analyzed for a number of key diagnostic measures including but not limited to the presence of red blood cells if stomach ulcerations were suspected and the presence of yeast or other concerning organisms.
- Endoscopic exams: As the behavior proved reliable, the tube was replaced by an endoscope, allowing for full visual examination of the trachea and stomach.

ULTRASOUND

One of the easiest behaviors to train marine mammals was teaching them to accept an ultrasound examination. The development and use of this behavior took longer to develop than other behaviors primarily due to lack of portable ultrasound equipment in the early years combined with the fact that pregnancies had not previously been monitored as closely or detected as early. The development of other behaviors, such as blood sampling, made it easier to monitor changes in progesterone levels, which naturally led to the desire to conduct ultrasound exams. Because this behavior is an extension of other tactile behaviors, often already being used for other reasons, the addition of training an animal to accept the application of gel and an ultrasound transducer to the routine was not difficult. These steps required gradual introduction of these new things over time and required gradual extension of the amount of time that an animal had to remain still. Many animals have been easily trained to remain still and allow an exam to continue for up to 20 minutes uninterrupted, far longer than was usually required.[18,25,26]

OTHER MEDICAL BEHAVIORS

As the skill set of marine mammal trainers grew and the helpfulness of trained medical behaviors became obvious, creative veterinarians, trainers, and animal care managers continued to push the limit of what was possible. Each year at marine mammal conferences and in marine mammal publications, there have been reports of new and unique veterinary behaviors being trained. A few examples are listed next:

- Urine samples: The early training of this behavior was accomplished as animals were taught to lay still and allow the trainer to put pressure on the bladder while another trainer or veterinarian collected the sample in a syringe as it was expressed.[9,27–29] This was quickly followed by putting the urination on cue; bladder pressure was no longer needed to elicit the desired response.[30–32] In a few facilities, trainers were even able to teach animals to accept insertion of a catheter to allow a more sterile urine sample to be taken.[33]
- Breath samples: Teaching the animals to forcefully exhale on cue and into a culture plate became commonplace and was useful in getting cultures of organisms in the animal's airway.[9,11,14]
- Morphometric measurements: As animals became more and more comfortable being handled and touched, it became far easier to get weights, lengths, girth, and any other important measurement.[10,11,13,34]
- Semen collection: As the focus on breeding efforts increased and the need to better understand reproductive processes grew; several facilities developed and perfected a variety of techniques for training males to present their penis and for collecting of semen samples. The earliest technique used included targeting the tip of the penis to a finger (through inserting the finger into the genital slit). Once the animal understood that the goal was to touch their penis to the finger, the finger would be gradually removed from the genital area, causing the animal's penis to become erect.[35,36] Another technique used was to simply watch for appropriate muscle movements in the genital region of the male and to reinforce the animal each time he or she offered the appropriate movement of the muscle, which would eventually lead to an erection. This later technique led to the discovery of several muscles that can be seen to move externally that are indicative of muscle movement within—by observing and reinforcing this movement, training animals for semen collection has proved more predictable and successful for many species of cetaceans.[37,38] Not as much work has been done with this behavior in pinnipeds.
- Artificial insemination: Most of these projects are done with the female out of the water and under some type of restraint. However, several facilities have successfully trained their females to remain in a ventral up position under behavioral

control to allow the insertion of a catheter and endoscope so that the insemination procedure can be accomplished without restraint.[35,39]

- Nasal swabs and nasal endoscopy: This particular behavior was first perfected with pinnipeds and later transitioned to its use with dolphins. Working around the animal's head can initially be uncomfortable for most animals; thus, it is often much later in an individual animal's learning that working around the nose or blowhole can be accomplished.[16,40]

- Saliva collection: Several studies have been conducted to compare information from a sample collected in a relatively passive manner, such as saliva sampling to samples that are more difficult to acquire such as blood collection. Although the information found in a saliva sample was not as useful as blood sampling, it was found to be a beneficial procedure for some animal health teams.[41]

- Throat cultures: In many cases, if an animal has been trained for stomach tube insertion, that behavior can be modified to become a way of getting a culture sample from an animal's throat.[16,18,28]

- Milk collection: As many facilities began to have breeding success, the ability to collect milk samples became on important behavior. Human milk pumps were adapted to fit over the mammary area of dolphins and the animals were trained to accept the sensation of the pressure from the suction of the pumping device. Once trained, this behavior was used to monitor nutritional content of milk as well as used to collect and store milk for future use.[28,30,42]

- Teeth brushing: Working around the mouth can take some time to train, because trainers and veterinarians must always be concerned about their own safety. As trust is developed between animal and trainer, behaviors around the mouth can get easier. However, even dangerous animals that must be trained in protected contact can safely be trained to have their teeth brushed. In these cases, the handle on the tooth brush may need to be much longer than normal to safely get inside the animal's mouth. The first step to the teeth brushing behavior is teaching the animal to open its mouth on cue, followed by acceptance of the brush and allowing the teeth to be touched by the brush. These first steps are relatively easy to train; often the difficult step is getting the animal comfortable with the taste of whatever dental solution or paste the veterinarian prescribes.[16,24,28]

- Fecal samples and rectal swabs: Getting a clean fecal sample from a marine mammal, especially a cetacean, can be difficult. In cetaceans, normal feces dissipate quickly and thus cannot usually be collected after the fact. The only way to get a fecal sample was usually through the insertion of a piece of clear rubber airline tubing into the anus. By teaching the animal to accept the insertion of these small tubes and gradually approximating the animal's tolerance of the tube going farther and farther up the rectum, a fecal sample could easily be collected. As this behavior was perfected, the logical next step was to substitute a culture swab for the tube and perform rectal swabs.[16,43]

- Positioning for radiographs: This behavior was first perfected with pinnipeds. Their ability to stay on dry land for long periods of time made it easier to teach them to lay down on or next to a radiographic plate. The 2 most challenging parts of this behavior are getting the animal comfortable with the large equipment needed to get the image and teaching the animal to remain motionless for long enough to get a clean image. Although positioning of cetaceans for radiographs takes a bit more creativity, trainers have had success in teaching the behavior with dolphins and whales as well.[16,24,44]

- Injection of medications: This behavior is an extension or variation to the blood-taking behavior; it is trained the same way. Once an animal is well trained, the behavior can be used for regular administration of injectable antibiotics if needed.[16,28] Additionally, some facilities have found ways to train animals for mild or passive restraint so that an injection can be accomplished more easily.[45]

- Eye and ear drops: This is yet another behavior requiring the trainer to work around the head. As long as care is taken to protect the trainers and the animal, many different behaviors around the head can be trained. Two of the most sensitive is acceptance of drops or ointment in the animal's eyes or ears. Because marine mammals live in a water environment, one of the important aspects of this behavior after teaching the acceptance of something being put into their eyes and ears is teaching them to keep their head out of the water for a prolonged period of time to give the medication time to take effect.[16,24,43]

- Nail trimming: This is not a behavior needed for cetacean care but can be useful in pinnipeds as well as penguins and otters, not to mention many terrestrial and avian species. In addition to the safety measures talked about previously, trainers doing the clipping need to be familiar with the anatomy of the nail to make sure that too much of the animal's nail is not clipped all at once. This can cause discomfort and cause the behavior to break down. By trimming in very small increments, the behavior is more easily maintained and the risk of causing discomfort for the animal is greatly reduced.[24]

TRANSITION TO OTHER SPECIES

The success of medical training with marine mammals and the advantages that were demonstrated in the health and well-being of the animals being trained prompted many zoos to take note and to begin exploring how this could be implemented in other species. The Association of Zoos and Aquariums invited IMATA to provide a special presentation about medical training at their annual conference in 1989.[46] In the years that followed, zoos began to hire supervisors, managers, and curators of training and enrichment; it had become evident that training was a key role in animal care and that skilled trainers needed to be a part of a good animal care team.[47] This eventually led to the creation of a new organization for zoological trainers called the Animal Behavior Management Alliance in 1999.[48] Through this organization and other professional organizations, the training of medical behaviors with many new species has been documented.

ANIMAL WELFARE

Certainly the most notable benefit from training has been the ways in which it has benefited animal welfare.[47,49] Training has proven to be a mechanism that reaches far beyond teaching an animal to participate in a medical behavior; it gives the caregiver the ability to provide greater opportunities for physical exercise and far more options for mental stimulation in the zoological environment.[50] These elements are what make training one of the key foundations to providing good animal care and ultimately provides for the animal's welfare. Trainers, managers, and veterinarians should not take training for granted and assume that training a medical behavior will be possible with every animal or that training is worth it "at all costs." Like most decisions, caregivers must weigh the benefits to the animal measured against the time and costs of implementation. Additionally, because so much of making an animal comfortable with medical procedures is related to taking the time to train procedures slowly, moving too quickly can be counter to providing excellent welfare; while taking the time to do it right can ensure good welfare. These factors must be considered when determining which medical behaviors each program chooses to train.[5]

SUMMARY

Training is an important key to improving animal care, and the marine mammal community has demonstrated this fact through its success in developing medical behaviors and techniques that have been transferred from species to species, even those not part of the marine mammal community. A few critical points follow:

- The use of positive reinforcement is essential to successful medical behavior training.
- There are many foundational behaviors that an animal must learn to be able to successfully learn and maintain medical behaviors.
- The training of some medical behaviors takes time; they cannot be rushed or the benefits of training will be lost.
- Medical behaviors must be practiced frequently to maintain their usefulness.
- Use the information learned from previous training of individual behaviors to aid in successful training with new animals and new species.

ACKNOWLEDGMENTS

The author would like to acknowledge and thank Joe Heyden of the Shedd Aquarium for his tireless hours of literature searches and for checking all the reference citations.

REFERENCES

1. Messinger C, McGinnis T. Marineland: images of America series. Charleston (SC): Arcadia Publishing; 2011.
2. Pryor K. Shaping. Lads before the wind. Waltham (MA): Sunshine Books; 2000. p. 21–42.
3. Pryor K. Dolphin training for everyone: the clicker revolution. Lads before the wind. Waltham (MA): Sunshine Books; 2000. p. 315–28.
4. Ramirez K. Husbandry. Animal training: successful animal management through positive reinforcement. Chicago (IL): Shedd Aquarium Press; 1999. p. 133–211.
5. Ramirez K. Husbandry training. In: Irwin M, Stoner J, Cobaugh A, editors. Zoo technology. Chicago (IL): University of Chicago Press; 2012, in press.
6. Benaroya M, Priest G, Ramirez K. Training, an essential part of every animal's care. In: Proceedings of the 27th Annual Conference of the International Marine Animal Trainers Association. Chicago (IL); 1999. p. 34–43.
7. Hurley J, Holmes N. A review of the psychological principles and training techniques associated with desensitization. Marine Mammals Public Display Res J 1998;3:16–26.
8. Sweeney J. Medical care and general husbandry practices. In: Proceedings of the International Marine Animal Trainers Association Conference. Redwood City (CA); 1978. p. 8–11.
9. Krames B. The conditioning of various behaviors for animal husbandry of killer whales. In: Proceedings of the 12th Annual Conference of the International Marine Animal Trainers Association. Rancho Palos Verdes (CA); 1984. p. 51–5.
10. Withrow R. Husbandry and training of Hawaiian monk seals (an endangered species) at the Waikiki Aquarium. In: Proceedings of the 12th Annual Conference of the International Marine Animal Trainers Association. Rancho Palos Verdes (CA); 1984. p. 11–8.

11. Sweeney J. The clinic's corner: medical procedures: the easy way. Soundings 1984;9(4):2.
12. Sweeney J. The clinic's corner: husbandry behaviors: making them work. Soundings 1987;11(2):7–8.
13. Ramirez K, Messinger D, Snyder C, et al. Husbandry and training of an orphaned bottlenose dolphin. In: Proceedings of the 15th Annual Conference of the International Marine Animal Trainers Association. New Orleans (LA); 1987. p. 67–74.
14. Sweeney J, Moderator. Husbandry behaviors: training, use, and maintenance. A panel discussion. In: Proceedings of the 17th Annual Conference of the International Marine Animal Trainers Association. Amsterdam, Netherlands; 1989. p. 113–33.
15. Messinger D, Marrin-Cooney D, Traxler A, et al. Trainer's forum: training voluntary husbandry behaviors in *Tursiops*. Soundings 1990;15(3):10–1.
16. Charfauros V. Trainer's forum: training husbandry behaviors with pinnipeds. Soundings 1990;15(1):16.
17. Antrim J. Trainer's forum: training a voluntary blood sample with a California sea lion. Soundings 1990;15(1):17.
18. Zeligs J, Costa DP. Trained complex veterinary procedures in Zalophus californianus at USSC Long Marine Lab. In: Proceedings of the 18th Annual Conference of the International Marine Animal Trainers Association. Chicago (IL); 1990. p. 183–9.
19. Shinder D. Separation and removal of marine mammals for medical examination. In: Proceedings of the 11th Annual Conference of the International Marine Animal Trainers Association. Apple Valley (MN); 1983. p. 93–102.
20. Litz C. Stretcher conditioning at the Living Seas. In: Proceedings of the 14th Annual Conference of the International Marine Animal Trainers Association. Vancouver (Canada); 1986. p. 48.
21. Skaar D. Stretcher training for handling whales and dolphins. In: Proceedings of the 15th Annual Conference of the International Marine Animal Trainers Association. New Orleans (LA); 1987. p. 35–8.
22. Desmond T. Tube insertion training of Orcinus orca and Tursiops truncatus. In: Proceedings of the 12th Annual Conference of the International Marine Animal Trainers Association. Long Beach (CA); 1984. p. 4.
23. Messinger D, Ramirez K. Trainer's forum: the training of stomach tube insertion with a bottlenose dolphin. Soundings 1987;11(2):5.
24. Sevenich M. Trainer's forum: training husbandry behaviors with pinnipeds. Soundings 1990;15(1):16.
25. Sweeney J. Diagnostic ultrasound – how do you make sense of the scratch? In: Proceedings of the 17th Annual Conference of the International Marine Animal Trainers Association. Amsterdam (Netherlands); 1989. p. 112.
26. Wells R, Luna R, Gifford T, et al. Ultrasonic blubber depth monitoring as a dolphin husbandry tool. In: Proceedings of the 20th Annual Conference of the International Marine Animal Trainers Association. Freeport (Grand Bahamas); 1992. p. 33.
27. Blasco D. Trainer's forum: training voluntary urine samples from dolphins. Soundings 1990;15(2):18.
28. Lacinak CT, Scarpuzzi M, Force D, et al. Husbandry training as a tool for marine mammal management: update. In: Proceedings of the 21st Annual Conference of the International Marine Animal Trainers Association. Kailua-Kona (HI); 1993. p. 13.
29. Blasco D. A fluke haul-out behavior develops increased desensitization techniques in overall husbandry success. In: Proceedings of the 21st Annual Conference of the International Marine Animal Trainers Association. Kailua-Kona (HI); 1993. p. 25.

30. Ramirez K. Husbandry behaviors for the care and treatment of a pregnant dolphin with kidney stones. In: Proceedings of the 24th Annual Conference of the International Marine Animal Trainers Association. Gold Coast (Australia); 1996. p. 17.

31. Baker J, Davis J, Granberry T, et al. Training urine collection on Atlantic bottlenose dolphins. In: Proceedings of the 28th Annual Conference of the International Marine Animal Trainers Association. Playa del Carmen (Mexico); 2000. p. 16.

32. Lenzi R. Operant conditioning and ultrasound together at work to successfully condition voluntary urine collection. In: Proceedings of the 28th Annual Conference of the International Marine Animal Trainers Association. Playa del Carmen (Mexico); 2000. p. 17.

33. De Souza R, Cardoso O, Lacave G, et al. Dolphin training for cystoscopy. In: Proceedings of the 23rd Annual Conference of the International Marine Animal Trainers Association. Las Vegas (NV); 1994. p. 19.

34. Messinger C, Messinger D, Dye G, et al. Determining morphometric accuracy in *Tursiops truncatus*. In: Proceedings of the 27th Annual Conference of the International Marine Animal Trainers Association. Chicago (IL); 1999. p. 24.

35. Keller K. Training Atlantic bottlenose dolphins (*Tursiops truncatus*) for artificial insemination. In: Proceedings of the 14th Annual Conference of the International Marine Animal Trainers Association. Vancouver (Canada); 1986. p. 22–4.

36. Schreib S, Smith TD, Burrows A. Erection training with a sexually aggressive dolphin from a vulnerable species: goals, concerns and methods. In: Proceedings of the 18th Annual Conference of the International Marine Animal Trainers Association. Chicago (IL); 1990. p. 211–5.

37. Acton D. Conditioning semen collection with a Pacific white-sided dolphin. In: Proceedings of the 29th Annual Conference of the International Marine Animal Trainers Association. Albuquerque (NM); 2001. p. 18.

38. Hudson JO. The training of semen collection for Tursiops truncatus, the Atlantic bottlenose dolphin. In: Proceedings of the 30th Annual Conference of the International Marine Animal Trainers Association. Orlando (FL); 2002. p. 21.

39. Im T, Chan S, Rayner C, et al. Artificial insemination in Tursiops truncatus aduncus. In: Proceedings of the 28th Annual Conference of the International Marine Animal Trainers Association. Playa del Carmen (Mexico); 2000. p. 24.

40. Marrin-Cooney D. Video recording the nasal passage of an echolocating dolphin. In: Proceedings of the 17th Annual Conference of the International Marine Animal Trainers Association. Amsterdam (Netherlands); 1989. p. 27–30.

41. Sullivan T. The conditioning of bottlenose dolphins, *Tursipos truncatus*, for collection of saliva. In: Proceedings of the 18th Annual Conference of the International Marine Animal Trainers Association. Chicago (IL); 1990. p. 20–3.

42. Komolnick T, Reddy M, Miller D, et al. Conditioning a bottlenose dolphin (*Tursiops truncatus*) for mil collection. In: Proceedings of the 20th Annual Conference of the International Marine Animal Trainers Association. Freeport (Grand Bahamas Island); 1992. p. 24.

43. Ramirez K, Hudson M, Takaki L. Initiation of a sea otter training program. Marine Mammals Public Display Res J 1996;2(1):43–9.

44. Massimi M, Horjus P, Strickland S, et al. Training a southern sea otter for voluntary radiographs. In: Proceedings of the 28th Annual Conference of the International Marine Animal Trainers Association. Playa del Carmen (Mexico); 2000. p. 27.

45. Stacy R, Messinger D, Dye, G, et al. Passive restraint training in Tursiops truncatus. In: Proceedings of the 25th Annual Conference of the International Marine Animal Trainers Association. Baltimore (MD); 1997. p. 28.

46. Pearson J, Sullivan T. Husbandry behaviors: a look at what is possible. In: Proceedings of the American Association of Zoological Parks and Aquariums Annual Conference. Pittsburgh (PA); 1989. p. 318.

47. Ramirez K. History of animal training. Animal training: successful animal management through positive reinforcement. Chicago (IL): Shedd Aquarium Press; 1999. p. 5–8.

48. Hellmuth H. What is ABMA? Available at: http://www.theabma.org/index.php?option=com_content&view=article&id=63:newsflash-2&catid=45:what-is-abma&Itemid=127. Accessed February 26, 2012.

49. Mellen J, Ellis S. Animal learning and husbandry training. In: Kleinman D, Allen M, Thompson L, et al, editors. Wild animals in captivity: principles and techniques. Chicago (IL): The University of Chicago Press; 1996. p. 88–99.

50. Ramirez K. What is training? Animal training: successful animal management through positive reinforcement. Chicago (IL): Shedd Aquarium Press; 1999. p. 8–12.

Using Operant Conditioning and Desensitization to Facilitate Veterinary Care with Captive Reptiles

Heidi Hellmuth, BS[a],*, Lauren Augustine, BA[a],
Barbara Watkins, MA[a], Katharine Hope, DVM[b]

KEYWORDS

- Reptile • Training • Operant conditioning • Desensitization

KEY POINTS

- In addition to being a large component of most zoological collections, reptile species are also becoming more and more popular as family pets.
- Reptiles have the cognitive ability to be trained in order to facilitate daily husbandry and veterinary care. Desensitization and operant conditioning can alleviate some of the behavioral and physiological challenges of treating these species.
- A survey of reptile training programs at zoos in the United States and worldwide reveals that there are many successful training programs being used in zoological settings to facilitate veterinary care and minimize stress to the animal.
- Many of the techniques being used to train reptiles in zoological settings are transferable to the exotic pet clinician. These techniques are useful for improving veterinary care in private herpetological collections and for the family pet.

INTRODUCTION

Many reptile species have become increasingly popular as pets. Exotic animal veterinarians are well aware of the impact that stress can have on their patients, and how that stress can impact both the quality of the examination and overall health of the animal. Utilizing operant conditioning techniques during veterinary procedures can decrease the stress associated with the visit and increase the effectiveness of the procedures. This article examines how different training and conditioning techniques

The authors have nothing to disclose.

[a] Department of Animal Programs, Smithsonian's National Zoological Park, 3001 Connecticut Ave, NW, Washington, DC 20008, USA; [b] Department of Animal Health, Smithsonian's National Zoological Park, 3001 Connecticut Ave, NW, Washington, DC 20008, USA
* Corresponding author.
E-mail address: hhellmuth@verizon.net

Vet Clin Exot Anim 15 (2012) 425–443
http://dx.doi.org/10.1016/j.cvex.2012.06.003
1094-9194/12/$ – see front matter Published by Elsevier Inc.

can facilitate improved veterinary care and management of reptiles in the home, at the exotic animal clinic, and in zoological settings.

REPTILE HEALTH—DISEASES, DIAGNOSTICS, AND THERAPIES
Common Diseases Seen in Reptiles

Captive reptiles can develop a variety of illnesses, ranging from infectious to neoplastic to husbandry-related. As with any species, a complete history and physical examination, with appropriate diagnostic testing, are essential to accurately diagnosing and treating the animal. A challenge with many exotic species is to understand and minimize stressors that can affect behaviors and physiologic parameters in order to obtain the most accurate diagnosis. This section will review common diseases of reptiles, examination and diagnostic testing, and how the stress during veterinary procedures can affect interpretation and treatment of animal illnesses.

The exotic practitioner very commonly encounters husbandry-related illnesses in reptiles, many of which are related to the precise environmental parameters (eg, temperature, humidity, ultraviolet exposure, substrate) and diet that these species require. Common husbandry-related problems seen in reptiles include dysecdysis, metabolic bone disease, obesity, vitamin deficiencies, traumatic abscesses, and stomatitis. A thorough examination of any reptile must require a complete investigation of its housing and diet, both current and historical, to detect or rule out husbandry-related disease.

Infectious diseases are also frequently encountered in captive reptile species, both in pets and in zoological collections. Of the infectious diseases, endo- and ectoparasite infections can be simplest to diagnose, requiring a positive identification from a fecal sample or skin sample, though other parasitic infections can necessitate more extensive testing (eg, radiographs or gastric biopsy). Bacterial, viral, or fungal infections can be slightly more challenging to diagnose; and usually require more extensive testing, including oral, nasal, or cloacal swabbing for polymerase chain reaction or culture, blood collection for culture, or serologies for identification of the etiologic agent.[1]

Finally, in addition to the reptile-specific husbandry and pathogen-related diseases, captive reptiles experience degenerative, metabolic, traumatic, or neoplastic diseases just as do nonreptile species. A thorough diagnostic examination must investigate all likely causes of disease.

Effects of Stress in Evaluating Animal Health

Reptiles can react to psychological or physical stress in ways that make it difficult to interpret behavior, examination findings, or laboratory values. Creating a less stressful environment is important for observing natural behaviors such as ambulation, head and eye movements, and response to stimuli. Stressed reptiles may display false symptoms of illness such as erratic behavior or feigning death, particularly seen in hognose snakes (Heterodon spp), and increased respiration rates have been seen in response to elevated corticosterone levels in western fence lizards (Sceloporus occidentalis).[2]

The physiological and physical stress that may occur during an examination can affect diagnostic results and potentially harm the animal. Studies have shown that exogenous administration of corticosteroids can cause hyperglycemia in certain lizard and snake species.[3–5] Decreased cholesterol content of liver, increased urea content of liver and kidney, and increased activity of glucose-6-phosphatase in the liver and kidney has been noted in lizards following corticosteroid administration.[4] However, the response to exogenous corticosteroids, and the production of endogenous steroids, can be seasonal for some species.[6,7] Exhaustive activity in laboratory crocodilians resulted in a significant decrease in blood pH and a significant increase in blood lactate levels,[8,9] suggesting that forceful restraint in an examination may alter blood chemistry. Interestingly, a study in painted turtles showed that when put in situations of forced anoxia, glucose and lactate levels rose; however, during recovery corticosterone levels rose as lactate fell, suggesting that steroids may play a role in lactate metabolism and clearance.[9] Additionally, handling alone can cause increased corticosterone levels which in turn can cause increased energy demands in already compromised patients.[10,11] Forceful restraint can lead to trauma (eg, fractures in an animal with metabolic bone disease or osteomyelitis) and some herpetofauna will drop their tails in response to stressful handling. Due to the physiologic and physical responses to stress, desensitizing captive reptiles to handling can be important in developing an ability to perform a successful examination, obtaining accurate diagnostics, and preventing injury to the animals.

The Reptile Examination

To minimize stress during the examination, the room or enclosure should be an appropriate temperature for the species in order to observe the animal's behaviors as normally as possible. External stimuli should be minimized, and if possible, species-specific items may be used to help the animal feel more comfortable (eg, chameleons may prefer to have a branch to hold on to during the examination).

The most important diagnostics in any reptile examination are a thorough history and a complete physical examination. History must include information on husbandry (substrate, lighting, humidity, temperature gradient), diet, exposure to other animals, where and when it was obtained by the owner, behavior, appetite, fecal and urate production, weight, and any other pertinent information related to the cause of the veterinary visit. Prior to handling the animal, practitioners should attempt to observe its activity, appropriateness, and ambulation. Latex gloves must be worn during the physical examination, and experienced handlers should be employed to ensure the animal is comfortable and thus maximize the diagnostic value of the exam. Most pet reptiles can be examined under manual restraint alone. However, some species or individuals may require additional restraint devices (such as tubes, poles, boxes, or protective gloves) or techniques (such as placing visual barriers or employing the vasovagal response) in order to minimize movement during the examination. Procedures usually performed in awake reptiles include blood samples for hematology, blood chemistry, and blood culture; fecal samples; oral, nasal, or cloacal swabs; aspirates; radiographs; and ultrasound. Diagnostics that require anesthesia include rigid or flexible endoscopy, advanced diagnostic imaging, and surgery.

Therapies and Monitoring

It is important to ensure that thorough records, including regular weight, feeding, and husbandry information, are maintained. The owner or keeper must be able to assess the animal's behavior, condition, and any physical abnormalities to note any changes. Correcting husbandry concerns is a top priority for treating both husbandry- and non–husbandry-related illness in reptiles. Sick reptiles should be kept at the high end of their temperature gradient in order to increase their metabolic rate and support the immune system. Humidity must also be carefully controlled depending on the disease—for example, high humidity may benefit animals undergoing dysecdysis, but may predispose an already compromised animal to secondary fungal infections. Diet adjustments may need to be made including offering different types of prey, or sometimes syringe or tube feeding or placing an esophageal feeding tube.

Systemic medications can be administered enterally or parenterally. Generally, orally administered medications are most desirable as owners can administer them at home, but oral drugs can be difficult to administer reliably in an effective time frame depending on the animal's feeding schedule and willingness to accept food and/or medication. Injectable medications are frequently administered subcutaneously, intra-muscularly, intravenously, or intracoelomically, and are usually uncomplicated in reptiles but do require increased veterinary attention to administer. Topical medications such as liquids, creams, or baths are also common therapeutics employed.

Most aspects of veterinary care, from diagnosis to treatment, can be facilitated with operant conditioning. Additionally, trainers, who are well-versed in observing animal behavior, are able to spot tiny changes in an animal's behavior,[12] which can be critical to detecting subtle signs that may indicate a veterinary problem. This article will review how training techniques can minimize stress and maximize veterinary care in captive reptiles.

REPTILE COMMUNICATION AND COGNITION
Reptile Communication Channels

Communication is defined as "the cooperative transfer of information from a signaler to a receiver."[13] Humans have very familiar ways of transferring information, intentions, and desires with other mammals. Verbal cues and hand gestures are used with great success when training other mammals that have acute vision and hearing. However, reptiles have modes of communication that are less familiar and require a different training approach. When training reptiles it is important to understand the specific species' communication channels. Generally speaking, communication in reptiles occurs visually, acoustically, tactilely, and chemically, with animals often relying on multiple methods to receive input simultaneously.[13]

Visual communication in reptiles can range from the movement of a specific body part to dramatic color displays. An obvious example of visual communication is a head bobbing display for courtship or territoriality in many species of lizard.[13] Body coloration and color change can be sexually dichromatic and are forms of visual communication.[14] In laboratory studies conducted on highly visual lizard species, females painted with male coloration elicited aggressive behavior from other males when placed in terraria, and similar responses were documented when males were painted with female coloration.[14] Specific snake species, such as king cobras (*Ophiophagus hannah*), are highly visual hunters that respond to prey movement. It has been suggested that tortoises seek out brightly colored vegetation in foraging for food[15] and crocodilians are known to be very visual predators.[16] Many species utilize courtship gestures, submissive postures, tail displays, and various signaling mechanisms in communication.[14]

Auditory communication is evident with various reptile species across many taxa, including vocal calls, bellowing, body parts being rubbed to produce a sound, and slapping the body against a specific surface, such as head slaps in water with crocodilians.[13] New research also indicates that snakes may in fact hear air-borne sounds.[17] There is even evidence that a nonvocal reptile, the Galápagos marine iguana (*Amblyrhynchus cristatus*) can hear and utilize the alarm call of the Galápagos mockingbird (*Nesomimus parvulus*) to respond with its own anti-hunter behaviors to their shared predator, the Galápagos hawk (Buteo galapagoensis).[18]

In tactile communication, an animal uses its body to rub, press, or hit another animal. In tortoises this manifests as neck biting, hindlimb stroking, chin rubbing, spur stroking, shell ramming, and biting[14]; caudocephalic and cephalocaudal waves are seen in snake courtship and are best described as contractions of movement against the female's body prior to copulation.[14] Snakes interpret ground-borne sounds through vibration transferred through the body to the skull,[19] in addition to air-borne sounds.[17] This concept of sensation through touch can be used in a training program. For example, tortoises will respond to neck rubs and tactile reinforcers and snakes can respond to cues that cause slight vibrations when training.

A primary mode of communication for many species of reptile is chemical signaling. Many species rely heavily on skin and cloacal secretions during mating. An experiment involving garter snakes (*Thamnophis sirtalis* and *T butleri*), where estrous females were covered with petroleum jelly to conceal signaling by skin secretions, showed that males that were once receptive were no longer interested in mating with the females.[20] Snakes and lizards have highly developed senses of smell that can be utilized in a training program; for example, an effective training method is to use a prey scent trail to train a snake to move when needed, taking advantage of a natural predatory behavior in the animal—seeking prey by scent—to accomplish a desired behavior with reduced stress (Janis Gerrits, Washington, DC, personal communication, January 2012).

Reptiles are a diverse group of animals that require varied training approaches to appeal to specific physiologic and behavioral tendencies or inclinations for each taxon. When approaching training opportunities with such a vast number of different species, the natural history, and communication channels of each should be studied and incorporated into the training plan.

Reptile Cognition

It is a common misconception that ectotherms lack cognitive abilities. Research has demonstrated that reptiles display behavioral complexity and have the ability to learn.[21–25] For example, behavioral complexity and play in a Komodo dragon (*Varanus komodoensis*) at the Smithsonian's National Zoo were documented by introducing a series of objects to the lizard. This study suggests significant cognitive abilities of this large, long-lived reptile, which has been trained at many zoological institutions to allow behavioral restraint for veterinary care. A related species, the black throated monitor (*Varanus albigularis*), has also shown cognitive and problem solving abilities, learning how to open a hinged door to gain access to food items.[26] Operant conditioning has been increasingly used with reptiles in zoological settings over the past 10 years[22,23,25,27–29] to facilitate veterinary care and more complex approaches reflecting reptile intelligence are being incorporated into training programs. For example, 4 adult Aldabra tortoises (*Geochelone gigantea*) learned to associate a clicker with food, to target, and then to hold still with their necks extended to the target to allow venipuncture of the jugular vein.[25] In another example, a Nile crocodile (*Crocodylus niloticus*) was taught to associate a whistle with food, then target and station on cue, which eventually allowed staff to obtain a weight and blood draw without sedation or restraint.[22] Studies in indigo snakes (*Drymarchon corais*) have shown that their rate of response to operant conditioning is similar to comparable studies of rats that had been trained to press levers or disc-pecking pigeons.[30]

Previously mentioned examples of reptilian cognitive abilities and training successes have focused on large animals that many veterinarians may never see in their offices. However, there are examples of smaller reptile species displaying cognition. Researchers at Duke University documented problem solving in the emerald anole (*Anolis evermanni*), where the animal demonstrated the ability to problem solve by removing a disc to gain access to a covered food item.[31] The test subjects also learned to discriminate between the target and a distracter disc placed in close proximity to the target, displaying cognitive abilities and behavioral flexibility comparable to many endothermic species. With documented case studies, new research emerging, and continued success in various reptile training programs in zoological settings, it is clear that reptiles have significant cognitive abilities.

REPTILE TRAINING
Benefits of Operant Conditioning

Behavioral training has many purposes and benefits for animals including physical exercise, mental stimulation, reducing stress, research, work and service functions, increased safety, cooperative behavior, and more. But one of the most important reasons for training animals is to better provide for the animals' physical and mental welfare.[32] And contrary to the beliefs of some, there are no boundaries as to which species can be trained.[33]

Veterinary care is an important part of a captive animal's life, and it is in the best interests of all involved to make the process as positive as possible. Stress can have adverse impacts on reptiles and as such should be minimized when possible. Studies on farm and laboratory animals show that handling for some veterinary procedures can be stressful, but if the animals learn to associate desired consequences with these interactions, the degree of fear responses they exhibit can be reduced.[34] This is certainly applicable to reptilian taxa, and should be considered when owning, housing, and treating any captive specimen.

Training has proved to be beneficial in mammals, producing more accurate diagnostic analysis for biochemical data. In rhesus monkeys (*Macaca mulatta*), cortisol levels were significantly higher when animals were trained versus restrained for blood collection.[35] Other research has shown reductions in stress hormones[36,37] and stereotypic behavior[38] as beneficial effects of training. Similar results have been described in bongo (*Tragelaphus euryceros*) with significantly reduced cortisol levels for crate-trained animals when restrained in the crate for 20 minutes,[39,40] close to baseline cortisol levels for resting cattle.[41,42] The bongo trained for restraint had lower creatine phosphokinase and glucose levels than animals immobilized by dart or pole syringe.[40] Livestock cared for by workers who build relationships (eg, patting, stroking, moving slowly) versus ones who use aversive interactions (eg, quick movements, shouting, hitting) showed reduced fear of humans.[43,44] Lab-housed stump-tailed macaques (*Macaca actdoides*) considered friendly by caretakers received more attention and interactions, were less disturbed by procedures, and were more likely to approach and accept food from caretakers.[45] And in a zoo study, reproduction in small exotic cats was more successful when keepers spent time interacting with the animals.[46] These studies are evidence that teaching animals to cooperate in their own health care can make life less stressful for both the animal and the trainer.[32]

Safety is a primary concern when working in close proximity to any animal. Both animals and people are at risk due to fear-based behavior. Animals showing fear responses can be dangerous animals.[47] They are more likely to injure themselves or their handlers than are animals that are not showing behaviors indicative of fear.[41,48,49] All vertebrates can learn to associate a fear response with certain stimuli.[50,51] Some animals learn to pair a fear response with the presence of the veterinarian.[47] Operant conditioning can also be used to reduce fear responses and pair positive reinforcers with the veterinarian and medical procedures. Training animals to cooperate with handling procedures helps reduce stress and accidents,[47] thus improving safety for humans and animals alike (**Box 1**).

Even with potentially dangerous animals such as venomous snakes, there are a variety of tools made specifically for working more safely with them, including hooks,

Box 1
Case Study 1: Caiman Lizard (Dracaena guianensis), Schönbrunn Zoo, Vienna, Austria

The caiman lizard is a large, semi-aquatic lizard from the Amazon River basin can reach at least 412 mm SVL (snout-vent length). These carnivorous reptiles spend time both in trees and in water, and hunt snails as their primary source of prey (Mesquita et al, 2006).

The Schönbrunn Zoo in Vienna, Austria received 2.2 caiman lizards from a breeding farm in Peru in August 2008, when the animals were 8–12 months of age. Once the animals were stable and eating consistently in an off exhibit area, they were moved to a large, 40 square meter enclosure; designed with many plants, rock walls, a river with a pond, and a variety of climbing structures. The lizards were fed their favorite food – apple snails – in two or three different locations throughout the enclosure.

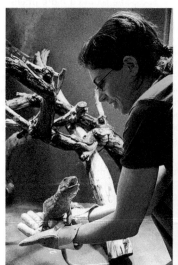
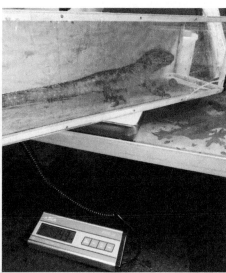
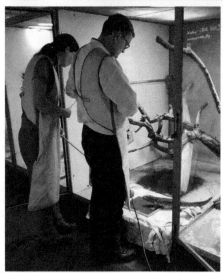

Left to right: Caiman lizard being desensitized to handling gloves, caiman lizard targeted into box and on scale, caiman lizard targeting onto x-ray cassette for radiographs. (*Courtesy of* Archiv Tiergarten Schönbrunn; *Data from* Mesquita DO, Colli GR, Costa GC, et al. At The Water's Edge: Ecology of Semiaquatic Teiids in Brazilian Amazon. J Herpetol 2006;40(2):221–9.)

After a short time in their new exhibit, a variety of management problems arose. One female lizard became quite dominant and aggressive towards the others, and was able to eat most of the snails; and was also the likely culprit in a tail injury received by the other female. One of the male lizards hid, probably in the rock wall, and wasn't able to be located for several weeks.

To help mitigate these problems, a behavioral training program was implemented, with an initial goal of being able to individually feed and check each animal regularly. A second goal was to desensitize the lizards to handling, because after each time the animals were caught up for any reason, they exhibited fear and stress behaviors for a long period afterwards.

Training began in a terrarium behind the scenes. Some individuals allowed keepers to approach closely enough to offer snails with tweezers, and some required more intensive training to get to this point. After spending some time pairing a clicker (as a bridging stimulus) with a snail, a target pole was introduced, and the lizards soon learned to touch and follow the target. Targeting was used to guide the lizards over a variety of different materials for desensitization, such as cloth, metal, wood, and leather; and they learned to follow the target through objects such as pipes and boxes, including into a transport crate. The desensitization training allowed the staff to begin touching and handling the lizards with heavy leather gloves without stressing the animals; and the targeting behavior also allowed keepers to train the lizards to go into a crate voluntarily. The crating behavior was useful for a wide variety of other management and veterinary behaviors, as the crate could easily be placed on a scale to obtain weights, and over an x-ray film cassette for radiographs. The lizards were also able to be targeted directly on to the film cassette for radiographs as well, which added flexibility in utilizing this diagnostic tool.

The training program has been very successful in helping to better and more safely manage this amazing species. The staff discovered that in addition to easier and less stressful handling, the lizards are now more relaxed in the presence of the keepers and they show less aggression to each other within the group.

tongs, shields, snake cans, and tubes.[52] Utilizing the proper tools in combination with operant conditioning techniques, it is possible to train many reptilian species regardless of their size or venomous nature (**Box 2**).

Utilizing Training in Veterinary Care

There are numerous behaviors that can be used to facilitate many aspects of veterinary care, from diagnosing the problem to administering treatment. Reptiles respond to operant conditioning, and training should be used to minimize stress and maximize the ability to medically evaluate and treat these animals. This section will focus on some of the more useful behaviors and their application to veterinary exams, and will review specific examples (Appendix 1) of how training and desensitization enable veterinary procedures with reduced stress.

Desensitization

"Desensitization is the process of getting an animal used to a new stimulus through gradual exposure to it. The stimulus may be people, other animals, noises, lighting, or anything the animal may perceive as new or frightening."[32] Desensitization can be trained with both active and passive methods. Passive desensitization is called habituation, where an animal gets used to new things on its own over time, without active involvement from a trainer and without pairing the association with reinforcement.[32] With this technique the animal needs to be able to choose to go near or interact with the new stimulus; it should not be forced into close proximity or it might result in increased fear responses.[53]

Box 2
Case Study 2: Nile crocodile (*Crocodylus niloticus*), Wildlife Conservation Society, Bronx Zoo, Bronx NY

The Nile crocodile is a large predator native to Africa, which can grow to lengths of 6 meters (Trutnau and Sommerland 2006). Likely because of their impressive size, Nile crocodiles are one of the most commonly kept crocodilian species in captivity. However, their size and physiology creates many challenges to maintaining them in captivity.

In response to these challenges, the Bronx Zoo utilized operant conditioning to facilitate examining and treating large crocodilians in captivity. A training program for an adult male Nile crocodile was initiated in May 2008 soon after his arrival. First a whistle bridge was conditioned; then a target behavior was trained. Initially mastering targeting in the water, the animal's potential was quickly seen and the keepers began opportunistically working him on land.

To take this training further, a protocol for blood draw training was drafted. But before this training could commence there were some safety concerns to be addressed. Entering the exhibit with an eight-foot Nile crocodile is dangerous, and facility modifications were completed to reduce the risks and safeguard the keeper and veterinary staff. The animal was slowly habituated to human presence in the exhibit and then desensitized to touch on his tail. With a combination of facility modifications for safety, desensitization to a variety of people and stimuli, and step by step operant conditioning techniques, the crocodile was able to be stationed on a scale and blood was successfully collected in March 2010.

The use of this training could have tremendous ramifications. By desensitizing this animal to touch as well as habituating him to human presence, veterinarians can safely approach this animal for physical exams, injury assessments and treatments. The collection of regular blood samples could allow veterinary staff the ability to further study crocodilian disease and treatment as well as document normal blood values for that animal and the species. In addition this behavior could possible allow for injectable treatments on this animal if necessary.

Data from Trutnau L, Sommerland R. Crocodilians: Their Natural History and Captive Husbandry. 1st edition. Frankfurt (Germany): Brahm AS; 2006.

Active desensitization, or counter conditioning, is a process where the new stimulus is paired with or followed by reinforcement to create a positive association with that stimulus.[32] Counter conditioning gives the trainer more control over the process and progress can frequently move at a more rapid pace than habituation. Both methods of desensitization can be beneficial in the training of cooperative behaviors for veterinary visits and examinations. The involvement of veterinarians in desensitization for veterinary visits and medical behaviors is critical. They are needed stimuli that will be present for procedures and should therefore be part of the training process. Other training includes desensitizing the animal to the equipment that will be used, the physical contact that is required for the exam, the duration of the procedure, and the number of people that need to be present.[32]

Taking the time to get animals used to and comfortable with the situations and equipment they might encounter in a veterinary visit can go a long way in making a more receptive and cooperative participant. The Denver Zoo routinely handles several species of non-venomous snakes to desensitize them to veterinary exams (Patricia Anderson, Denver, CO, personal communication, January 2012). At the Schönbrunn Zoo in Austria, keepers desensitized their Caiman lizards (*Dracaena sp*) to leather gloves and veterinary equipment to prepare them for veterinary visits (Dr Eveline Dungl, Vienna, Austria, personal communication, January 2012) (**Box 3**). At the North Carolina Zoo, keepers desensitized an American alligator to a sit under a nebulizer for pneumonia treatments (Chris Shupp, Asheboro, NC, personal communication, February

> **Box 3**
> **Case study 3: False water cobras (*Hydrodynastes gigas*), Smithsonian's National Zoo, Washington, DC**
>
> False water cobras are rear fanged, venomous colubrids that occur naturally in South America (Greene, 1997). They are large semi-aquatic snakes, feeding mostly on frogs and fishes (Bels, 1987; Strüssmann & Sazima, 1993). Their biology makes them great exhibit animals, utilizing aquatic, terrestrial, and arboreal features in the exhibit at the Smithsonian's National Zoo.
>
> Three juvenile false water cobras are exhibited together in the Reptile Discovery Center. When multiple snakes are housed together, feeding the animals in a manner that avoids conflict, aggression, and possible ophiophagia (eating of the other snakes) is of top concern and usually results in the animals being separated during feeding. Typically, venomous snakes are hooked off-exhibit into a secure holding container (referred to as canning) for routine exhibit maintenance and feedings. False water cobras are known to be very active, vigorous feeders which can be a challenge, but in this circumstance, proved to be a wonderful training opportunity. To date, each individual animal has been successfully trained to follow a scented target pole into an off-exhibit holding can for each feeding session. By scenting a target stick, animals are enticed to follow the target stick and willingly enter the can. The animal is rewarded for this behavior with mice left in the bottom of the can.
>
> This has proven to be an effective tactic used while performing routine husbandry practices, and many future uses as well. It is now a very easy task to weigh and manipulate the animals into any number of containers for safe handling, allowing for veterinary assessment and possible treatments. Additionally, this training likely reduces the stress for animals and keepers by minimizing hooking efforts, as well as decreasing the time it takes to separate and move animals.
>
> *Data from* Refs.[65–67]

2012); and at the Fort Worth Zoo, a Komodo dragon has been desensitized by the keeper staff and is trained to allow a mask to be placed on its head for anesthesia during veterinary exams (Diane Barber, Fort Worth, TX, personal communication, February 2012).

Animals that are regularly handled for routine procedures are likely to experience less stress when captured for an uncommon procedure.[54] As one trainer put it, "We teach the animals to help us take care of them ... we teach the animals that going to the vet is a game and we play that game every single day, whether a vet is there or not. And those 'games' include numerous veterinary or cooperative behaviors. To the animal, it's just part of the training session."[55]

Tactile Desensitization

An important behavior to teach animals for a veterinary examination is to accept tactile stimulation.[56] While not every species or individual is amenable to this technique, animals that have been taught to accept being touched will be easier to manage. And, although some animals may seem to solicit petting or tactile interactions, this does not automatically mean they will do so for medical procedures. Desensitization is a critical component to establishing reliable tactile interactions and is helpful for husbandry procedures.[32] Tactile desensitization training should begin with parts of the body where the animal is most receptive to touch, and the animal should never be surprised by the touch.[57] Animals should be made aware that a touch is going to occur, either through a verbal signal or other sensory cue. This strategy can help reduce potential aggressive behavior from a surprised animal and help prevent damaging the trust between the trainer and animal.[56]

At the Smithsonian's National Zoo, daily habituation and tactile desensitization has become a key component in the medical care of an adult male Komodo dragon. As part of this animal's management, cleaning and exhibit maintenance are done in the morning, and feeding in the afternoon. Every morning, when the animal's body temperature is lower and it is less active, the keeper completes the needed exhibit work and then engages the animal with tactile interaction. Over time, the lizard has become habituated to this routine, and the veterinary team is able to enter the animal's enclosure and obtain radiographs without heavy restraint or sedation (Janis Gerrits, Washington, DC, personal communication, January 2012).

Targeting/Stationing

Basic behaviors such as targeting and stationing are excellent ways to position and manipulate an animal in order to better assess health concerns. A target is an object that an animal is taught to touch, follow, or go to. It can be a ball on the end of a stick, a hand, a straw, spoon, or any object that the animal can perceive and is safe to use.

Once an animal understands the target behavior concept, targeting can be used as a tool in training many other behaviors. It can be part of an active desensitization program, where an animal follows a target to, and even on or through, novel items (Dr Eveline Dungl, Vienna, Austria, personal communication, January 2012). It can be used to teach an animal to go onto a scale, into a crate, and countless other behaviors. For example, the Colchester Zoo used the targeting behavior to move their crocodiles and Komodo dragons for examination, to obtain weights, blood draws, ultra sounds, nail trims, and to apply topical medication (Jez Smith, Essex, United Kingdom, personal communication, January 2012). These behaviors are sometimes initiated with baiting or luring—where the animal is shown food or food is put on/in the desired item (ie, crate or scale) to entice the animal to approach. Baiting, while a useful training tool, can be problematic if the animal needs to be fasted for medical reasons but requires food in order to perform a task.[56] Targeting is a much more effective tool in these instances.

Stationing is an offshoot of the targeting behavior; it refers to training an animal to go to a specific item or location, and tells the animal where it is expected to be for a behavior or during a training session.[32] When training a reptile for veterinary care, the station can be a familiar item that carries reinforcement value in an unfamiliar environment. For example, if an animal is trained to station on a piece of Astroturf, this can easily be brought to the veterinarian's office and put on a scale or exam table for stationing during the exam.

Both stationing and targeting are foundation behaviors that are at the core of a good training program. If they are trained to fluency, they offer the animal the opportunity to present a behavior that has a strong history of positive reinforcement in a veterinary setting. This can potentially lead to a more relaxed and cooperative patient in an unfamiliar environment.

Box/Squeeze/Tube

Training an animal to enter a mobile shift or squeeze box can reduce stress for transportation and can be useful for basic husbandry. This can be a permanent or temporary attachment to the animal's enclosure and should be dark, warm, or in some way attractive to the reptile. Animals can be fed in the shift box, so that the reptile has a positive association with the shift. At the Buffalo Zoo, black tree monitors (*Varanus beccarii*) have been trained to station in a plastic container for weighing (Penny Felski and Illa Caira, Buffalo, NY, personal communication, February 2012).

The shift box can be a clear, acrylic squeeze cage so that the patient can be visually inspected by the veterinarian, and so that the animal can be restrained into a smaller space to receive injections, facilitate anesthesia, or accomplish blood draws. Several institutions have animals trained to enter clear containers for veterinary exams, including poison dart frogs (*Dendrobates* sp) at Disney's Animal Kingdom (Mindy Sommer, Lake Buena Vista, FL, personal communication, January 2012), green mamba (*Dendroaspis angusticeps*) at the Brookfield Zoo (Tim Sullivan, Brookfield, IL, personal communication, January 2012), and Komodo dragons at the Toronto Zoo (Nicole Presley, Toronto, Canada, personal communication, February 2012), and Singapore Zoo (Sarah Chin, Singapore, personal communication, February 2012).

Another tool is a snake immobilization tube that, when combined with operant conditioning, can be a highly effective method for safely handling and examining venomous species. Operant conditioning can be used to train the snake to enter the tube voluntarily rather than with force. One method utilized at the Riverbanks Zoo was to use the targeting behavior to train a king cobra to enter a tube. This, however, proved more difficult than anticipated so keepers had to initially bait, or used food to entice the animal into the tube.[28] Baiting allowed the animal handlers to desensitize and eventually target train the snake into the tube.[28]

CHALLENGES IN TRAINING REPTILES

Although training is a useful tool for facilitating veterinary care, there are many challenges that must be addressed when training reptile species. It is important to remember the animal's health and welfare is top priority, and training should not commence if it compromises the animal's health.

Overfeeding

The food requirements of reptiles vary depending on the specimens' size, age, temperature, activity,[58] and reproductive status.[59] As ectotherms, reptiles are characterized by low metabolic rates and high conversion efficiencies.[60] Overfeeding is a commonly seen problem with amateur herpetologists.[61,62] Obesity can increase the likelihood of liver disease, cardiac disease, arthritis, and renal disease.[58] When designing a training program it is imperative to keep the animal's diet consistent and appropriate for the species and individual.

Frequency of Feeding

The time and frequency of feeding reptiles is of significant importance when training. Some species will readily eat any time, while others are strictly nocturnal or diurnal feeders.[63] Additionally, many species will fast for weeks or months in the wild as an adaptation to the natural environment or reproductive status and this can persist in captivity.[63] The frequency in which animals are trained and fed will directly affect the success of a training program. Most mammals eat several times a day, making the potential training regimen much more intensive than that of a reptile that can consume as little as 1 meal a month in captivity. In order to maximize training sessions with these animals, it is imperative to use every feeding session as an opportunity to train the animal. Caregivers can increase the frequency of training and still maintain the animal's caloric intake by offering smaller food items that, cumulatively, are the equivalent to one large meal. Feeding several small items or portions instead of one large meal can increase training approximations during each individual session.[29] Each species' natural feeding behavior should be taken into consideration when a dietary change is made for training purposes. For example, grazers such as tortoises can easily have their diet split up and offered to them throughout the day, but this strategy may not be as feasible with all reptilians.

Food Delivery

Understanding how reptiles perceive the world is important when feeding a captive specimen. Reptiles use several senses simultaneously when feeding; in particular olfactory, visual, and thermal cues. When approaching an enclosure with food, the olfactory cue has likely been delivered and the next cue is the visual presentation of food. Reptiles have varying degrees of vision, snakes for the most part have relinquished an emphasis on visual cues[19] where lizards are often utilizing vision for prey and mate selection.[64]

A challenging aspect of training reptiles is delivering the food reinforcer safely and in a timely manner, especially when working with venomous species and/or animals known for aggressive behavior. This can then be exacerbated when multiple animals are in an enclosure together. Hand delivery of food poses risks. Hand delivery requires the trainer's hand to get within close proximity of the reptiles' mouth. If tossing the food, there is a chance the animal may miss the food item and/or see the movement of the trainer's hand and perceive that quick motion as the food. Both of these examples can cause injury or adversely affect training outcomes. Many tools are available to effectively deliver food to animals when training including tongs, feeding sticks and forceps.

If an animal is hesitant to approach the caregiver, proximity training can be an effective method of slowly desensitizing the animal to a person's presence during feeding. This training, combined with the different lengths of tongs available, can ease the animal into the new feeding regime.

When utilizing feeding tools the delivery is often slower, providing the animal with a number of cues or signals that food is coming, making reinforcing the desired behavior challenging. The olfactory cue, in combination with a slow delivery of food, can elicit an aggressive feeding response that may inadvertently be reinforced. This type of feeding response can be minimized by training the animal to sit at a station where feeding will occur.

Tools, especially tongs, are often used for cleaning, feeding and manipulating the animal or cage furniture. When a tool is used repeatedly to feed an animal, the animal may form an association between it and the food. When used for other purposes, the tongs will likely elicit a feeding response even when not being used for feeding. Additionally an animal can sustain an injury during tong feeding if it is overly motivated to feed. Animals that are new to tong feeding tend to bite the tongs and abrade in and around the mouth. This can be avoided by using padded tongs, and reinforcing and shaping a calm feeding behavior.

A feeding stick is another option for delivering food reinforcers. A dowel rod or other similar item can easily be fashioned into a feeding stick by whittling one end into a dull point. This point can be used to skewer food onto the end of the rod, without posing a danger to the animal. Another tool option is forceps, which are used much like tongs and come in a variety of lengths. These are appropriate for aquatic species and species that eat small prey. They will allow delivery of the food while maintaining a safe and comfortable distance, without overpowering the food with a large delivery tool. Forceps might also minimize the feed response to a multipurpose tool like tongs.

Environmental Conditions

The environmental conditions that are ideal for keeping reptiles can prove to be yet another challenge for training. Reptile enclosures are usually small, are kept at higher temperatures, and are uniquely designed to the species being exhibited. For example, an enclosure might require a significant amount of perching for a particular species or a large pool of water for a semi-aquatic species. When attempting to train a reptile, especially a small lizard or snake, the door must often remain open during the session. When working with quick moving species, minimizing or eliminating animal escapes needs to be a priority. To avoid escapes from enclosures, it is best to move the animal to a more appropriate training space, or when this is not possible, training the animal to station away from the door can increase safety and reduce the risk of an escape.

Reptiles may be housed individually, in pairs, or in social groups. Housing animals together may cause dominance hierarchies amongst the animals, and more dominant animals to over-eat while submissive animals receive less food. Dominant animals will generally be more easily trained. Forming a relationship with the more submissive animal can be difficult, especially with the dominant animal(s) present. Removing a reptile from the enclosure can help focus on training goals with the other animal. At the Smithsonian's National Zoo a keeper trained a very active and food motivated Mertens' water monitor (*Varanus mertensi*) to follow a target into a holding container in order to isolate and train the animal's exhibit mate (Janis Gerrits, Washington, DC, personal communication, January 2012).

Paradigm Shift

While the use of operant conditioning training to facilitate management and veterinary care has gained more widespread acceptance in recent years, its application with reptiles and amphibians has lagged behind that of their mammal and avian counterparts. This could be due to the ease with which many reptiles can be involuntarily picked up or restrained for examinations, or it could be related to the lack of reptile and amphibian training models for caregivers to learn from. For those who work with or own mammals or birds, they can look to an abundance of examples of training; from dog training for obedience and agility to an array of animal shows at zoos and aquariums with a wide variety of taxa. Even when reptiles are involved in these types of shows and demonstrations, they are generally carried or held, and rarely are shown being trained to exhibit active or natural behaviors during these programs. A paradigm shift is needed, with keepers, owners, and veterinarians learning about and embracing the benefits of operant conditioning as a critical component in the care of reptiles and amphibians.

Even once this paradigm shift occurs, a challenge still remains. Operant conditioning is a skill set that must be learned; reptile owners and veterinarians need to make an effort to learn this useful technology to benefit their animals. While there are many wonderful training resources available, there are none dedicated to the specific challenges of working with reptiles and amphibians. Fortunately, training is training, and the art and science of animal training is transferable to any species, any animal.[53]

SUMMARY

Reptiles are capable of responding to operant conditioning and should have training programs incorporated into their captive husbandry. Of the many benefits training affords, the most important is its use in diagnosing and treating an ill animal. Veterinary clinicians should inform their clientele about the benefits operant conditioning can provide for the reptiles in their care.

ACKNOWLEDGMENTS

We would like to thank everyone who responded to our surveys and shared their training experiences for use in this article: Patricia Anderson, Denver Zoo; Diane

Barber, Fort Worth Zoo; Jason Brock, Zoo Atlanta; Sarah Chin, Singapore Zoo; Dr Eveline Dungl, Schönbrunn Zoo; Penny Felski and Illa Caira, Buffalo Zoo; Janis Gerrits, Smithsonian's National Zoological Park; Justin Graves, Smithsonian's National Zoological Park; Raelene Hobbs, Melbourne Zoo; Jack M. Jewell, Mandalay Bay Aquarium; April Martin, National Aquarium in Baltimore; Darren Minier, University of California at Davis; Shannon Osterholm, Blank Park Zoo; Nicole Presley, Toronto Zoo; Nelly Rivera, Theater of the Sea; Chris Shupp, North Carolina Zoo; Jez Smith, Colchester Zoo; Mindy Sommer, Disney's Animal Kingdom; Jake Steventon, Tennessee Aquarium; Tim Sullivan, Chicago Zoological Society; and Kevin Torregrosa, St Augustine Alligator Farm.

REFERENCES

1. Jacobson E. Infectious diseases and pathology of reptiles. Boca Raton (FL): CRC Press; 2007.
2. Durant SE, Romero LM, Talent LG, et al. Effect of exogenous corticosterone on respiration in a reptile. Gen Comp Endocrinol 2008;156:126–33.
3. Miller MR, Wurster DH. Further studies on the blood glucose and pancreatic islets of lizards. Endocrinology 1958;63:191–200.
4. Jacob V, Oommen OV. A comparison of the effects of corticosterone and cortisol on intermediary metabolism of *Calotes versicolor*. Gen Comp Endocrinol 1992;85: 86–90.
5. Houssay BA, Penhos JC. Pancreatic diabetes and hypophysectomy in the snake *Xenodon merremii*. Acta Endocrinol 1960;35:313–23.
6. Gist DH. Effects of mammalian ACTH on liver and muscle glycogen levels in the South American Caiman (*Caiman scleraps*). Gen Comp Endocrinol 1972;28:413–9.
7. Tyrell CA, Cree A. Relationships between corticosterone concentration and season, time of day and confinement in a wild reptile (Tuatara, *Sphenodon punctatus*). Gen Comp Endocrinol 1998;110:97–108.
8. Seymour RS, Bennett AF, Bradford DF. Blood gas tensions and acid-base regulations in the salt water crocodile, *Crocodylus porosus*, at rest and after exhaustive exercise. J Exp Biol 1985;118:143–59.
9. Keiver KM, Weinberg J, Hochachka PW. The effect of anoxic submergence and recovery on circulating levels of catecholamines and corticosterone in the turtle, *Chrysemys picta*. Gen Comp Endocrinol 1992;85:308–15.
10. Cash WB, Holberton RL, Knight SS. Corticosterone secretion in response to capture and handling in free-living red-eared slider turtles. Gen Comp Endocrinol 1997;108:427–33.
11. Dunlap KD, Wingfield JC. External and internal influences on indices of physiological stress. I. Seasonal and population variation in adrenocortical secretion in free-living lizards, *Sceloporus occidentalis*. J Exp Zool 1995;271:36–47.
12. Grandin T. Animals in translation. New York: Scribner; 2005.
13. Vitt LJ, Caldwell JP. Herpetology. An introductory biology of amphibians and reptiles. 3rd edition. Burlington (MA): Elsevier; 2009.
14. Carpenter CC, Ferguson GW. Variation and evolution of stereotyped behavior in reptiles. Part I. Survey of stereotyped reptilian behavioral patterns. In: Gans C, Tinkle DW, editors. Biology of the reptilia, vol. 7. London: Academic Press; 1977. p. 335–404.
15. Pellitteri-Rosa D, Sacchi R, Galeotti P, et al. Do Hermann's tortoises (Testudo hermanni) discriminate colours? An experiment with natural and artificial stimuli. Ital J Zoo 2010;17:481–91.

16. Webb G, Manolis C. Introduction to crocodilians. In: Australian crocodiles. Sydney (Australia): New Holland Publishers; 1998. p. 11–35.
17. Christensen CB, Christensen-Dalsgaard J, Brandt C, et al. Hearing with an atympanic ear: good vibration and poor sound-pressure detection in the royal python, *Python regius*. J Exp Biol 2012;215:331–42.
18. Vitousek M, Adelman J, Gregory N, et al. Heterospecific alarm call recognition in a non-vocal reptile. Biol Lett 2007;3:632–4.
19. Greene HW. Snakes: the evolution of mystery in nature. Berkeley (CA): University of California Press; 1997.
20. Noble GK. The sense organs involved in the courtship of Storeria, Thamnophis and other snakes. Bull Am Museum Nat Hist 1937;73:673–725.
21. Bustard HR. Rapid learning in wild crocodiles (*Crocodylus porosus*). Herpetologica 1968;24:173–5.
22. Augustine L. Husbandry training with an exceptional South African crocodile. ABMA Wellspring 2009;10:2–3.
23. Augustine L. Putting training to work in a large animal capture. ABMA Wellspring 2010;12:36–7.
24. Burghardt GM. Learning processes in reptiles. In: Gans C, Tinkle DW, editors. Biology of the reptilia, vol. 7. Bagneux: Academic Press; 1977. p. 555–681.
25. Weiss E, Wilson S. The use of classical and operant conditioning in training Aldabra tortoises (*Geochelone gigantea*) for venipuncture and other husbandry issues. J Appl Anim Welfare Sci 2003;6:33–8.
26. Manrod JD, Hartdegen R, Burghardt GM. Rapid solving of a problem apparatus by juvenile black-throated monitor lizards (*Varanus albigularis albigularis*). Anim Cogn 2008;11:267–73.
27. Gaalema DE, Benboe D. Positive reinforcement training of Aldabra tortoises (*Geochelone gigantea*) at Zoo Atlanta. Herpetol Rev 2008;39:331–4.
28. Vause K, Jones H. Training royalty at Riverbanks Zoo and Garden. ABMA Wellspring 2009;10:15–7.
29. Hellmuth H, Gerrits J. Croc in a box: crate training an adult male gharial. ABMA Conference Proceedings. San Diego (CA): Phoenix (AZ); 2008.
30. Kleinginna P. Operant conditioning of the Indigo snake. Psychon Sci 1970;18:53–5.
31. Leal M, Powell BJ. Behavioral flexibility and problem-solving in a tropical lizard. Biol Lett 2012;8:28–30.
32. Ramirez K. Animal training: Successful animal management through positive reinforcement. Chicago (IL): John G. Shed Aquarium; 1999.
33. Hosey G, Melfi V, Pankhurst S. Zoo animals: behaviour, management, and welfare. New York: Oxford University Press; 2009.
34. LeNeindre P, Bolvin X, Boissy A. Handling of extensively kept animals. Appl Anim Behav Sci 1996;49:73–81.
35. Reinhardt V. Working with rather than against macaques during blood collection. J Appl Anim Welfare Sci 2003;6:189–97.
36. Dettmer EL, Phillips KA, Rager DR. Behavioral and cortisol responses to repeated capture and venipuncture in *Cebus apella*. Am J Primatol 1996;38:357–62.
37. Elvidge H, Challis JRG, Robinson JS, et al. Influences of handling and sedation on plasma cortisol in rhesus monkeys (*Macaca mulatta*). J Endocrinol 1976;70:325–6.
38. Priest GM. Training a diabetic drill (*Mandrillus leucophaeus*) to accept insulin injections and venipuncture. Lab Prim Newsl 1991;30:1–4.
39. Grandin T. Habituating antelope and bison to cooperate with veterinary procedures. J Appl Anim Welfare Sci 2000;3:253–61.

40. Phillips M, Grandin T, Graffam W, et al. Crate conditioning bongo (*Tragelaphus eupycerus*) for veterinary and husbandry procedures at Denver Zoologicai Gardens. Zoo Biol 1998;17:25–33.
41. Alam MG, Dobson H. Effect of various veterinary procedures on plasma concentrations of cortisol, luteinizing hormone and prostaglandin E2 metabolite in the cow. Vet Rec 1986;118:7–10.
42. Grandin T. Assessment of stress during handling and transport. J Anim Sci 1997; 75:249–57.
43. Hemsworth PH. Human-animal interactions in livestock production. Appl Anim Behav Sci 2003;81:185–98.
44. Boivin X, Lensink J, Tallet C, et al. Stockmanship and farm animal welfare. Anim Welf 2003;12:479–92.
45. Waitt C, Buchanan-Smith HM, Morris K. The effects of caretaker-primate relationships on primates in the laboratory. J Appl Anim Welfare Sci 2002;5:309–19.
46. Mellen JD. Factors influencing reproductive success in small captive exotic felids (*Felis spp.*): a multiple regression analysis. Zoo Biol 1991;10:95–110.
47. Grandin T. Safe handling of large animals. Occup Med 1999;14:195–212.
48. Ames DR, Arehart LA. Physiological response of lambs to auditory stimuli. J Anim Sci 1972;34:994–8.
49. Boandle KE, Wohlt JE, Carsia RV. Effect of handling, administration of a local anesthetic and electrical dehorning on plasma cortisol in Holstein calves. J Dairy Sci 1989;72:2193–7.
50. LeDoux JE. Emotion, memory and the brain. Sci Am 1994;271:50–7.
51. LeDoux JE. The emotional brain. New York: Simon and Schuster; 1996.
52. Altimari W. Venomous snakes: a safety guide for reptile keepers. Society for the Study of Amphibians and Reptiles; St Louis, Missouri; 1998. p. 1–24.
53. Stafford G. Zoomility: keeper tales of training with positive reinforcement. An iReinfore.com Book; 2007.
54. Kreger MD, Mench JA. Physiology and behavioral effects of handling and restraint in the ball python (*Python regius*) and the blue-tongued skink (*Tiliqua scincoides*). Appl Anim Behav Sci 1993;38:323–66.
55. Davey P. Whales with fur: how to train any animal using dolphin training techniques. Flagler Beach (FL): Ocean Publishing; 2004.
56. Hellmuth H. Training 101. Smithsonian's National Zoological Park animal training manual. Washington, DC: Smithsonian; 2008.
57. Hellmuth H, Anderson C, Mello S, et al. For the birds: raptor training in a wildlife education program. Am Anim Trainer Magazine 2000.
58. Hackbarth R. Reptile diseases. Neptune City (NJ): TFH Publications; 1990.
59. Lillywhite H, Gatter R. Physiology and functional anatomy. In: Warwick C, Frye F, Murphy J, editors. Health and welfare of captive reptiles. New York: Chapman and Hall; 1995. p. 24.
60. Pough FH. The advantages of ectothermy for tetrapods. Am Nat 1980;115: 92–112.
61. Frye F. Husbandry, medicine and surgery in captive reptiles. Bonner springs Kansas: Veterinary Medicine Publishing; 1973. p. 140.
62. Warwick C. Reptilian disease in relation to artificial environments, with special reference to ethology. Int Colloq Path Med Reptiles Amphib 1991;4:107–19.
63. Donoghue S, Langenberg. Nutrition. In: Mader D, editor. Reptile medicine and surgery. Philadelphia: WB Saunders; 1996. p. 148–73.
64. Eric RP, Laurie JV. Lizards: windows to the evolution of diversity. Berkeley (CA): University of California Press; 2003. p. 333.

65. Bels V. Observation of the courtship and mating behavior in the snake Hydrody-nastes gigas. J Herpetol 1987;21(4):350–2.
66. Greene HW. Snakes, the evolution of mystery in nature. Los Angeles (CA) and London: University of California Press; 1997.
67. Strüssmann C, Sazima I. The assemblages of the Pantanal at Poconé western Brazil: faunal composition and ecology summary. Studies on Neotropical Fauna Environment 1993;28:157–68.

APPENDIX 1: EXAMPLES OF TRAINED BEHAVIORS FOR FACILITATING VETERINARY PROCEDURES IN REPTILE SPECIES FROM ZOOLOGICAL INSTITUTIONS WORLDWIDE

Institution	Species	Behaviors
Blank Park Zoo, IA	Aldabra tortoise, Geochelone gigantea	Target (weights, moves), Mouth open (oral exam) Desensitization (blood draws, diagnostic imaging, eye drops, eye pressure test, weights, foot exam)
Buffalo Zoo, NY	Black tree monitor, Varanus beccarii	Shift/Plastic container (weights, visual exam, diagnostic imaging)
Chicago Zoological Society-Brookfield Zoo, IL	American alligator, Alligator mississippiensis	Eye drops
	Green mamba, Dendroaspis angusticeps	Shift container (anesthesia, exams)
Colchester Zoo, United Kingdom	Komodo dragon, Varanus komodoensis	Station/Desensitization (diagnostic imaging, blood draws, nail trims, topical medications, weights)
	Crocodiles (various sp)	Target (exam)
Disney's Animal Kingdom, FL	Dart frogs, Dendrobates sp	Station (exam, weights)
Denver Zoo, CO	American alligator, Alligator mississippiensis	Station (reduce aggression)
	Various species	Station/Desensitization (exam)
Fort Worth Zoo, TX	Komodo dragon, Varanus komodoensis	Desensitization (anesthesia)
	Water/yellow tree monitor, Varanus sp	Target/Desensitization (exam), Crate (exam, moves) Target (exam), Station (exam,
	Indian gharial, Gavialis gangeticus	oral medications)
Mandalay Bay, NV	Komodo dragon, Varanus komodoensis	Target (exam, moves), Desensitization (nail trims), Crate (diagnostic imaging, exam, blood draws) Target (exam, moves), Crate
	Crocodiles/sea turtles (various sp)	(diagnostic imaging, exam, blood draws)
Melbourne Zoo, Australia	Aldabra tortoise, Geochelone gigantea	Target (weights), Desensitization (exam, blood draws, topical medications, diagnostic imaging, mouth inspection)

Riverbanks Zoo, SC	King cobra, *Ophiophagus hannah*	Shift/Tube (exam)
Schönbrunn Zoo, Austria	Morlett's crocodile, *Crocodylus moreletii*	Target (moves)
	Giant tortoise (various sp)	Target (moves, weights), Desensitization (exam)
	Caiman lizard, *Dracaena guianensis*	Crate (weight, diagnostic imaging), Desensitization (handling with gloves)
Sedgwick County Zoo, KS	Aldabra tortoise, *Geochelone gigantea*	Target (weights), Station/ Desensitization (blood draws)
Singapore Zoo, Singapore	Komodo dragon, *Varanus komodoensis*	Target (exam, moves), Desensitization (exam, diagnostic imaging)
Smithsonian's National Zoo, DC	Poison dart frogs, *Dendrobates sp*	Target (move to increase UVB intake)
	Indian gharial, *Gavialis gangeticus*	Crate (moves)
	Aldabra tortoise, *Geochelone gigantea*	Target (weights), Station (cooperative feeding)
	Komodo dragon, *Varanus komodoensis*	Desensitization (exam, diagnostic imaging)
	False water cobra, *Hydrodynastes gigas*	Target (shift off exhibit)
Theater of the Sea, FL	American alligator, *Alligator mississippiensis*	Target (moves, exam), Lift feet (exam, topical medications), Station (weights)
Toronto Zoo, Canada	Komodo dragon, *Varanus komodoensiss*	Shift/Crate (exam, nail trims, diagnostic imaging)
	Dwarf crocodile, *Osteolaemus tetraspis*	Shift (exam)
	Nile monitor, Varanus *niloticus*	Shift (exam)
	Chinese softshell turtle, *Pelodiscus sinensis*	Target (exam)
	American alligator, *Alligator mississippiensis*	Target (move, exam)
	Nile softshell turtle, Trionyx *triunguis*	Target (exam, weights), Desensitization (shell scrubs, topical medications, exam, crate)
UC Davis, CA	Snakes, tortoises, lizards (various sp)	Desensitization (restraint, exam, injections, diagnostic imaging, anesthesia)
Wildlife Conservation Society-Bronx Zoo, NY	Nile crocodile, *Crocodylus niloticus*	Target (exam), Station (exam, weights), Desensitization (exam, blood draws, zip-tie on snout)
Zoo Atlanta, GA	Aldabra tortoise, *Geochelone gigantea*	Target (weight, exam)
	Komodo dragon, *Varanus komodoensis*	Station (on wire mesh for nail trims)

Training Techniques to Enhance the Care and Welfare of Nonhuman Primates

Margaret Whittaker, BS*, Gail Laule, MA

KEYWORDS

- Animal training • Positive reinforcement • Animal welfare • Negative reinforcement
- Nonhuman primate training

KEY POINTS

- Nonhuman primates are excellent subjects for the enhancement of care and welfare through training.
- The application of positive reinforcement techniques to specific aspects of the management of captive nonhuman primates spans a wide range of species, social contexts, and housing situations (eg, laboratories, zoos, and sanctuaries).
- There is an increased interest from regulatory and accrediting agencies to insure improved conditions for captive nonhuman primates, apparent by the various standard guidelines, accreditation standards, and protocols available for the 3 primary types of nonhuman primate holding facilities.
- PRT is an invaluable component of captive animal management when it is used to enhance husbandry and medical care, mitigate aggression and increase affiliative behaviors and improve social management, reduce fear and anxiety, and enhance environmental enrichment programs; all contributing to an overall improvement in psychological well-being.

INTRODUCTION

Nonhuman primates are excellent subjects for the enhancement of care and welfare through training. The broad range of species offers tremendous behavioral diversity, and individual primates show varying abilities to cope with the conditions of captivity, which differ depending upon the venue and housing situation. In 1987, the Animal Welfare Act mandated that facilities housing nonhuman primates must provide for their psychological well-being; positive reinforcement training (PRT) has achieved wide recognition as a valuable tool for contributing to that objective.

The application of positive reinforcement techniques to specific aspects of the management of captive nonhuman primates spans a wide range of species, social

The authors have nothing to disclose.
Active Environments, Inc, 7651 Santos Road, Lompoc, CA 93436, USA
* Corresponding author.
E-mail address: indu22@earthlink.net

Vet Clin Exot Anim 15 (2012) 445–454
http://dx.doi.org/10.1016/j.cvex.2012.06.004
vetexotic.theclinics.com

contexts, and housing situations (eg, laboratories, zoos, and sanctuaries). Conditions for captive nonhuman primates vary widely depending on the situation. Housing in laboratory facilities may include small cages with a single individual, pair, or group housing, and corrals with large social groups. Zoos have social groupings of differing sizes, emphasizing natural behavior, public display, education, and reproduction. Sanctuaries typically have nonbreeding groups, which may consist of multiple species and varying numbers of individuals, and are not regularly on public display. In every venue, regardless of the institution's mission, a primary objective is to provide excellent care while addressing animal welfare and minimizing stress. Positive reinforcement training improves care and reduces stress by enlisting a primate's voluntary cooperation with targeted activities, including husbandry, veterinary, and research procedures. It is also used to improve socialization, reduce abnormal behaviors, and increase species-typical behaviors.[1–4] Environmental enrichment programs can be enhanced and expanded when PRT is applied.

There is an increased interest from regulatory and accrediting agencies to insure improved conditions for captive nonhuman primates, apparent by the various standard guidelines, accreditation standards, and protocols available for the 3 primary types of nonhuman primate holding facilities. Laboratory facilities are held to standards outlined in the "Guide for the Care and Use of Laboratory Animals" (2011),[5] which recommends that "Habituating animals to routine husbandry or experimental procedures should be encouraged whenever possible as it may assist the animals to better cope with a captive environment by reducing stress associated with novel procedures or people. In most cases, principles of operant conditioning may be employed during training sessions, using progressive behavioral shaping, to induce voluntary cooperation with procedures" (p. 64–5). In a recent 2010 report, of site visits to chimpanzee facilities in the United States, The Office of Laboratory Animal Welfare (OLAW) also supported the notion that PRT may help in reducing stress and concluded that when safe and feasible nonhuman primates should be afforded positive reinforcement training opportunities.[6]

The Association of Zoos and Aquariums (AZA) Animal Care Manuals (ACM) specify training and enrichment techniques to provide for improved care, welfare, and management of captive nonhuman primates. In the 2010 Chimpanzee ACM,[7] it is stated that "the use of positive reinforcement training as an animal care and management tool offers many benefits for chimpanzees and staff. One of the greatest benefits is to gain the voluntary cooperation of the chimpanzees in husbandry, veterinary, and research procedures. The fear and stress associated with these procedures, as well as the need for restraint and anesthesia can be significantly reduced. Greater choice and control can be provided to trained chimpanzees, contributing to their psychological well-being."[8] And it continues with further discussion regarding specific behaviors that can be trained through PRT: "using operant conditioning techniques, chimpanzees can be desensitized to frightening or painful events, such as receiving an injection, so that the event becomes less frightening and less stressful."[8] Voluntary cooperation reduces the need for physical restraint and/or anesthesia, and the accompanying risks associated with those events.[9,10]

The In Press Guenon Care Manual states that guenons "should be trained with positive reinforcement techniques for the routine modification of behavior to achieve management, husbandry, veterinary, and research behaviors, enhance socialization, facilitate introductions, and augment enrichment opportunities. Animal positioning should be achieved through the use of targets; animals should not be pushed, pulled, or coerced for routine training activities. Routine husbandry practices should include: shifting animals for activities such as daily cleaning, enrichment, exhibit maintenance, training animals to approach the cage front for close visual inspection of entire body, and presenting various body parts for both keepers and veterinary staff. Guenons should be trained to present for various types of injections (e.g. IM for anesthesia, intradermal for Tb testing, etc.), and because they are prone to developing diabetes; individuals tending towards this condition should be trained to voluntarily accept a subcutaneous injection in order to administer insulin. If any of these injections cannot be trained, guenons should be trained to enter a squeeze cage and accept squeeze restraint to facilitate treatments or procedures."[11]

Sanctuary housed primates, depending on the sanctuary, are held to standards that dictate the use of PRT. Chimpanzees housed in federally funded facilities must comply with the Standards of Care for Chimpanzees Held in the Federally Supported Chimpanzee Sanctuary Systems: Final Rule (Federal Register).[12] Section 9.6 Animal Care, Well-Being, Husbandry, Veterinary Care, and Euthanasia, (b) (iv) states that, "Many chimpanzees can be trained through positive reinforcement to cooperate with a variety of veterinary and chimpanzee care procedures. Efforts must be made to develop or maintain this capability for chimpanzees housed in the sanctuary to the extent possible. Trainers must use currently acceptable practices that do not include physical punishment." In (c) (xi), it is stated that "the sanctuary must minimize the use of physical and chemical restraint. Chimpanzees in the Sanctuary shall be trained to permit certain procedures with minimal or no restraint. Such procedures may include injections, dosing or other treatments, and cage-side health observations." Some apes may be trained to accept a manual injection for chemical immobilization, thus avoiding the stress of darting.[12]

The Global Federation of Animal Sanctuaries, a global nonprofit organization that verifies and provides an accreditation process for sanctuaries, has put forward the following standards for great apes and monkeys that pertain to handling and the use of certain techniques: "Where possible and appropriate, Positive Reinforcement Training is used to minimize the need for chemical immobilization and to reduce stress during procedures."[13,14] With appropriate training, many procedures can be performed cooperatively and without anesthesia, such as examination of body parts, treatment of superficial injury, heart rate monitoring — even EKGs and blood draws." And GFAS goes on to describe that aversive techniques should be avoided by saying, "Physical abuse, deprivation of food or water, aversive spraying with a hose, and other forms of negative reinforcement or punishment-based training are never used to train, shift or otherwise handle great apes."[14]

Clearly, PRT has become a recognizable component of enlightened captive animal management; with the greatest benefits seen in 4 main areas:

1. Improved husbandry and medical care through voluntary cooperation by the animals in a wide array of procedures
2. Enhanced social management and opportunity through training techniques that increase affiliative behaviors and decrease aggression
3. Improved psychological well-being through desensitization techniques that directly address fear and discomfort
4. Improved environmental enrichment programs by expanding options for enrichment strategies.

HUSBANDRY AND VETERINARY PROCEDURE TRAINING

There are many published articles on the benefits of PRT in gaining the voluntary cooperation of primates in husbandry and medical procedures. Since 1984, these authors alone have written over 25 different papers, chapters, and conference presentations on the subject.[8,15–22] Husbandry training facilitates routine husbandry and management practices, including: quick and reliable movement among all enclosure spaces[22] thorough visual exam of all individuals, and desensitizes animals to "routine" procedures, such as water supply checks, provisioning of food and enrichment, etc, that some nonhuman primates may find frightening. Veterinary training typically includes desensitization to fear inducing procedures such as injections, venipuncture for blood sampling, urine collection, and visual exams by veterinary staff. When trained to voluntarily cooperate in these procedures, animals have a choice in how the procedure will be carried out, rather than having to submit to anesthesia or physical restraint.[9,10,23]

With greater accessibility to more cooperative animals comes the opportunity to initiate preventive medicine practices and to explore techniques previously seen as less practical for routine use. Included are training for assisted reproduction techniques such as ultrasound and tube insertions for artificial insemination[24,25] and semen collection[26]; disease testing and health care practices such as Tb test administration; oral and some dental care; administration of oral and/or injectable medications and vaccinations; and wound treatment.[8,27–29] Voluntary cooperation in husbandry and veterinary procedures significantly reduces an animal's level of stress,[4,30–32] and it also causes less disruption for the entire group, by reducing the need to separate an individual in order to accomplish a task.[33,34]

With positive reinforcement methods proven to facilitate husbandry and veterinary care for captive primates, it is increasingly difficult to defend the use of negative reinforcement or escape/avoidance techniques to achieve these same goals. Subjectively, one can compare the behavior of a primate calmly accepting an injection to that of an agitated animal racing around the cage to avoid the dart gun. Objectively, one can compare the number of anesthetic events required to collect blood from an adult chimpanzee who cooperates voluntarily (none) to the number required to collect blood from an untrained animal (1 per blood sample). Both the subjective and the objective assessments make a strong case for the positive impact husbandry and veterinary training can have on an animal's well-being.

SOCIALIZATION

Many species of primates can be challenging to maintain in species-typical social groupings in captivity. Common problems include high levels of aggression and submission, serious wounding during introductions[35] and a lack of appropriate social skills. Objectives for training to improve the socialization of primates include (a) meeting the social needs of all group members, (b) reducing aggression and submission to acceptable levels, (c) increasing prosocial and affiliative behaviors, (d) facilitating the introduction of new animals to each other or into an existing group, and (e) gaining access to all individuals within the group. Positive reinforcement training offers specific methods to achieve each of these objectives.

Target Training

Targeting can elicit both gross and fine movements and teach animals to hold a position or location. Greater access to all individuals within the group is available when all group members will come to, go to, and stay at targets. The stationing of dominant animals lessens the possibility that they will interfere when subordinate animals receive food, enrichment, or medical attention.

Shifting Between Enclosures

Training animals to shift quickly and reliably and at any time of day, ensures the safety of the staff and the animals, and facilitates sound husbandry practices, including provisioning of regular and frequent enrichment strategies, enclosure maintenance, emergency preparedness, and ease of access to animals for training and veterinary procedures, etc. It also allows reinforcement of the group for moving simultaneously. Such reinforcement may promote a more cohesive group, which responds collectively toward a common goal.

Separation

Separation and temporary isolation of group-housed primates for management or veterinary purposes can cause undue stress for all members of the group and may trigger problems during the reintroduction of separated individuals. Training animals to separate voluntarily, as individuals or as subgroups, can facilitate the movement of animals into and out of the group and minimize the stress of separation. Voluntary separations also provide subordinate animals the occasional chance to escape the pressures of social housing. For species that are difficult to reintroduce following brief or more extended separations (eg, for veterinary procedures and recovery), reintroductions are made easier when voluntary separations are trained because the group is accustomed to and accepting of this practice. Calm separations can yield calmer reintroductions.[21]

Cooperative Feeding

Cooperative feeding is a technique used to enhance positive social behavior and reduce agonistic behavior in many species, including a variety of primates.[1,2,8,9,36–38] Rummel[39] suggests that aggression is an acquired, instigated, maintained, and modified behavior. Success in satisfying one's wants or needs will reward aggression, and if nonaggressive behavior is less successful in achieving satisfaction, aggression will increase. Dominant nonhuman primates receive reinforcement, both in the wild and in captivity, for managing the groups they lead, monitoring other group members, and acting as sentries. Many caregivers of captive animals have used subterfuge and distraction when attempting to provide subordinate animals with food, enrichment, or other desirable resources. However, these techniques actually exacerbate aggression, causing dominant animals to become more vigilant in order to maintain control of the desirable resources. In captivity, aggressive interactions can have serious consequences if group members are unable to escape the aggressors.

Cooperative feeding conforms to operant conditioning theory, which states that the consequences of a behavior determine whether it will recur.[40] Cooperative feeding is a specific technique wherein the dominant animal is carefully and purposefully reinforced for allowing the subordinate animal to receive a resource (typically food, attention from caregiver or trainer, or enrichment). This technique requires that the trainer reinforce the dominant animal for behavior that is cooperative rather than aggressive, thus strengthening cooperative behaviors. When consistently and skillfully applied, cooperative feeding will yield 2 shifts in the animals' behaviors: (a) the dominant animal's aggressive behavior when the subordinate receives valuable resources (food, enrichment, attention), and (b) the subordinate animal becomes less fearful and more willing to accept these resources that were previously refused in the presence of the dominant individual(s).

It is important to note that when cooperative feeding is used, the dominant animal's position in the hierarchy is not diminished. In fact, quite the opposite is achieved. Dominant animals are reinforced for allowing subordinates to have resources, and thus maintaining their position of dominance. They are typically provided with a higher quality or magnitude of reinforcement for allowing the subordinate to have something of lesser quality. Therefore, it becomes worthwhile for the dominant animal to allow the subordinate to have something in order to be reinforced with a preferred food item.

Gentle Touch and Proximity

"Gentle touch and proximity" behaviors are those that teach the concepts of touching gently and being close to another. This is introduced to the animals by first teaching the individual to touch the target gently. Directing this behavior toward another animal facilitates proximity (for which all animals are reinforced) and can elicit behaviors such as touching, grooming, mounting, and breeding.[37] Gentle touch may be especially helpful in managing introductions, encouraging affiliative behaviors, and decreasing abnormal levels of affiliation.[41] Desmond and Laule[42] reported positive results using this technique during the introduction of a silverback gorilla to a group of adult females, infants, and 1 hand-raised juvenile female. Additionally, in the first study examining the effects of socialization training, Cox[38] documented increases in all forms of affiliative behaviors after gentle-touch training sessions with a group of drills (Mandrillis leucopheus).

Collaborative Training

The authors use the term "collaborative training" to describe the latest concept in socialization training. This concept involves rewarding collaborative efforts in order to train animals to work together toward a common goal. The technique began with the training of cetaceans to perform group show behaviors requiring a coordinated effort, and it involves reinforcing the animals as a group. Therefore, if even 1 animal fails to perform the behavior to criterion, the group may not receive reinforcement.

Purposefully using behaviors that require animals to share a common goal to create social ties may enhance overall socialization. At one oceanarium, during a group "high bow" behavior, a hydrophone recorded vocalizations from multiple bottlenose dolphins during their underwater swim, then 1 single voice just before all the animals broke the surface of the water at the same time (T. Desmond, personal communication, May 16, 2006). Group-behavior training seemed to result in the formation of alliances between dolphins from different subgroups that then began to socialize more with each other outside of training and show times (W. Philips, personal communication, May 20, 2006). Similar results might be possible with primates, using such collaborative behaviors as retrieving an object too cumbersome for one animal to handle, passing objects between or among animals, and procuring desired food items under conditions requiring cooperation.

ADDRESSING FEAR AND DISCOMFORT

Forthman and Ogden[43] have cautioned animal managers never to presume, without supporting data, that animals have become habituated to routine procedures and handling. Their concern stems from studies on primates in laboratories, conducted nearly 20 years ago by Line and Markowitz and their colleagues.[44,45] These studies found prolonged alterations in heart rates and cortisol levels after such routine procedures as cage cleaning. In 1950, Hediger[46] suggested that fear of humans could be 1 trait that predisposes some species to poor captive welfare. Therefore, it is reasonable and logical to conclude that reducing fear in captive animals would improve their welfare.[47,48]

Desensitization

Desensitization is a very powerful, versatile, and valuable training technique for reducing anxiety when an animal demonstrates fear or discomfort associated with a particular event, person, situation, location, or object.[1,18] This training process pairs positive reinforcers with the frightening event or object. Establishing a direct relationship between the fear-inducing stimulus and positive reinforcers causes the fear to diminish over time. In 1 study, Clay and colleagues[48] demonstrated that desensitization was more effective at reducing fear in laboratory housed macaques compared to other experimental conditions. The rate of stress-related behaviors and cringing behaviors directed towards humans were reduced, as well as the duration of cringing directed toward humans.

The necessity of desensitizing an animal to all aspects of a veterinary procedure is apparent. An animal will not cooperate voluntarily if a procedure induces fear. Analyzing the physiological responses to voluntary and involuntary injections in chimpanzees, Lambeth and colleagues[4] found that cortisol was significantly higher in the involuntary condition and hypothesized that the voluntary condition reduced anxiety by giving the animal greater choice and control.

Desensitization may also provide significant assistance in managing social behaviors. For example, Brain and Benton[49] divided aggression into categories such as self-defensive behaviors and parental-defensive behaviors, and Moyer[50] characterized types of aggression as fear-induced, territorial, and maternal. These descriptions share a common thread of fear, discomfort, uncertainty, and apprehension. In the previously cited gorilla introduction carried out by Desmond and Laule,[42] the use of cooperative feeding and desensitization techniques with both the females and the silverback helped achieve a peaceful outcome, showing that desensitization can, in fact, successfully reduce the potential for aggressive behavior by addressing social stimuli which might otherwise produce fear.

ENHANCED ENVIRONMENTAL ENRICHMENT PROGRAMS

Environmental enrichment has been defined as "an animal husbandry principle that seeks to enhance the quality of captive animal care by identifying and providing the environmental stimuli necessary for optimal psychological and physiological well-being."[51] Enrichment can be divided into various categories including physical environment, choice gradients, manipulatable objects, feeding, sensory stimuli, social environment, occupational enrichment, and human interaction. Training can have an impact on each of these categories. Animals can be trained to use the entire physical environment and choice gradients, such as vertical spaces, when, for example, they do not fully utilize the enclosure. Manipulatable objects can be changed multiple times per day, providing improved enrichment opportunity and novelty, if animals are trained to quickly and reliably move between enclosures or on and off exhibit. Feeding enrichment, such as novel foods, can also be given throughout the day when animals readily move between areas. The use of complex feeding devices offers animals the opportunity to work at acquiring and processing their food; such devices greatly increase the amount of time spent in appetitive behaviors. Occupational enrichment offers animals the chance to "work for a living." Training is enriching and challenges animals to think. Since participation is voluntary, training is believed to be fun for animals.

SUMMARY

To date, the use of positive reinforcement training techniques with nonhuman primates has a fairly lengthy history and an impressive list of documented benefits. In fact, it is difficult to conceive of a convincing argument against the use of such training to achieve voluntary cooperation in husbandry and veterinary procedures, to enhance socialization and decrease aggression in these highly social animals, to reduce fear and anxiety associated with many aspects of captivity, and to enhance environmental enrichment programs. Because PRT is an affective tool that offers very real options for addressing the adverse consequences of captivity, every facility caring for nonhuman primates should integrate training strategies into its management systems and teach training techniques to its staff.

REFERENCES

1. Laule G, Bloomsmith M, Schapiro S. The use of positive reinforcement training techniques to enhance the care, management, and welfare of primates in the laboratory. J Appl Anim Welf Sci 2003;6(3):163–73.
2. Schapiro SJ, Bloomsmith MA, Laule GE. Positive reinforcement training as a technique to alter nonhuman primate behavior: quantitative assessments of effectiveness. J Appl Anim Welf Sci 2003;6(3):175–88.
3. Young RJ, Cipreste CF. Applying animal learning theory: training captive animals to comply with veterinary and husbandry procedures. Anim Welfare 2004;13: 225–32.
4. Lambeth SP, Hau J, Perlman JE, et al. Positive reinforcement training affects hematologic and serum chemistry values in captive chimpanzees (Pan troglodytes). Am J Primatol 2006;68:245–56.
5. National Research Council. Guide for the care and use of laboratory animals. 8th edition. Washington, DC: National Academies Press; 2009.
6. OLAW. Report on site visits to chimpanzee facilities and associated resources to aid grantee institutions. NOT-OD-10–121. Bethesda (MD): National Institutes of Health; 2010.
7. AZA Ape TAG. Chimpanzee (Pan troglodytes) care manual. Silver Springs (MD): Association of Zoos and Aquariums; 2010.
8. Laule GE, Whittaker M. The use of positive reinforcement techniques with chimpanzees for enhanced care and welfare. In: Brent L, editor. The care and management of captive chimpanzees. San Antonio (TX): American Society of Primatologists; 2001. p. 243–66.
9. Bloomsmith MA. Chimpanzee training and behavioral research: a symbiotic relationship. In: Proceedings of the American Association of Zoological Parks and Aquariums (AAZPA) Annual Conference. Toronto (Canada): AAZPA; 1992. p. 403–10.
10. Reinhardt V. Training nonhuman primates to cooperate during handling procedures: a review. Anim Technol 1997;48:55–73.
11. AZA Old World Monkey TAG. Guenon (Cercopithecus spp, Allenopithecus nigroviridis, Erythrocebus patas, Chlorocebus spp, and Miopithicus talapoin) care manual. Silver Springs (MD): Association of Zoos and Aquariums; 2012.
12. Rules and Regulations. Part 9.6 animal care, well-being, husbandry, veterinary care, and euthanasia. In: Federal Register 2008;73(198), Standards of care for chimpanzees held in the federally supported sanctuary system.
13. Bennet J. Standards for animal care of old world primates, version august 2011. Global Federation of Animal Sanctuaries (GFAS); 2011.
14. Bennet J. Standards for animal care of great apes, version august 2011. Global Federation of Animal Sanctuaries (GFAS); 2011.
15. Laule GE. Behavioral and husbandry intervention in the case of a hybrid Tursiops sp. Proceedings. In: Desmond TJ, editor. Proceedings of the International Marine Animal Training Association (IMATA) Annual Conference. Long Beach (CA): IMATA; 1984. p. 23–9.
16. Laule GE, Desmond TJ. Use of positive reinforcement techniques to enhance animal care, research, and well-being. In: Bayne K, Kreger M, editors. Wildlife

mammals as research models: in the laboratory and field. Bethesda (MD): Scientists Center for Animal Welfare; 1995. p. 53–9.

17. Laule GE, Whittaker M. The use of positive reinforcement techniques in the medical management of captive animals. Proceedings. In: Baer CK, editor. Proceedings of the American Association of Zoo Veterinarians (AAZV) and American Association of Wildlife Veterinarians (AAWV) Joint Conference. Omaha (NE): AAZV; 1998. p. 383–7.

18. Laule GE, Whittaker M. Enhancing nonhuman primate care and welfare through the use of positive reinforcement training. J Appl Anim Welf Sci 2007;10(1): 31–8.

19. Laule GE. The use of positive reinforcement training techniques to enhance the care, management, and welfare of primates in the laboratory. J Appl Anim Welf Sci 2003;6(3):163–74.

20. Whittaker M. Positive reinforcement training to enhance the care and welfare of captive animals [abstract]. In: Proceedings Joint Meeting of the Canadian Association of Laboratory Animal Science (CALAS) and the Association Canadienne Pour la Science des Animaux de Laboratoire (ASCAL). Montreal (Canada): CALAS/ASCAL; 2006.

21. Whittaker M. Training nonhuman primates in zoos. In: Proceedings of the American Veterinary Medical Association, presented at Annual Conference. Atlanta, GA. 2010.

22. Veeder CL, Bloomsmith MA, McMillan JL, et al. Positive reinforcement training to enhance the voluntary movement of group-housed sooty mangabeys (Cercocebus atys atys). J Am Assoc Lab Anim Sci 2009;48:192–5.

23. Reichard T, Shellabarger W. Training for husbandry and medical purposes. In: Proceedings of the American Association of Zoological Parks and Aquariums (AAZPA) Annual Conference. Toronto: AAZPA; 1992. p. 396–402.

24. Desmond TJ, Laule GE, McNary J. Training for socialization and reproduction with drills. In: Proceedings of the American Association of Zoological Parks and Aquariums (AAZPA) Annual Conference. Wheeling (WV): AAZPA; 1987. p. 435–41.

25. Logsdon S, Taylor S. Use of operant conditioning to assist in the medical management of hypertension in woolly monkeys. In: Proceedings of the Association of Zoos and Aquariums (AZA) Western Regional Conference. Louisville (KY): AZA; 1995. p. 96–102.

26. Perlman JE, Bowsher TR, Braccini SN, et al. Using positive reinforcement training techniques to facilitate the collection of semen in chimpanzees (Pan troglodytes). Am J Primatol 2003;60(Suppl 1):77–8.

27. Bayrakci R. Injection training lion tailed macaques. In: Animal Keepers' Forum (AKF) 2003;30(12):503–12.

28. Perlman J, Thiele E, Whittaker MA, et al. Training chimpanzees to accept subcutaneous injections using positive reinforcement training techniques. Am J Primatol 2004;62(Suppl 1):96.

29. Schapiro S, Perlman J, Thiele E, et al. Training nonhuman primates to perform behaviors useful in biomedical research. Lab Anim (NY) 2005;34(5):37–42.

30. Loehe R. Benefits of positive reinforcement training program with bonobos, Pan paniscus. In: Proceedings of the American Association of Zoos and Aquariums (AZA) Regional Conference. Louisville (KY): AZA; 1995.

31. Reinhardt V. Improved handling of experimental rhesus monkeys. In: Davis H, Balfour A, editors. The inevitable bond: examining scientist-animal interactions. Cambridge (United Kingdom): Cambridge University Press; 1992. p. 171–7.

32. Videan E, Fritz J, Murphy J, et al. Training captive chimpanzees to cooperate for an anesthetic injection. Lab Anim (NY) 2005;34(5):43–8.
33. Reinhardt V, Cowley D. In-homecage blood collection from conscious stump tailed macaques. Anim Welfare 1992;1:249–55.
34. Stone AM, Bloomsmith MA, Laule GE, et al. Documenting positive reinforcement training for chimpanzee urine collection. Am J Primatol 1994;33:242.
35. Erwin J. Aggression in captive macaques: interactions of social and spatial factors. In: Erwin J, Maple TL, Mitchell G, editors. Captivity and behavior: primates in breeding colonies, laboratories and zoos. New York: Van Nostrand Reinhold; 1979. p. 139–71.
36. Bloomsmith M, Laule G, Thurston R, et al. Using training to modify chimpanzee aggression during feeding. Zoo Biol 1994;13:557–66.
37. Desmond T, Laule G, McNary J. Training for socialization and reproduction with drills. In: Proceedings of the American Association of Zoological Parks and Aquariums Annual Conference. Bethesda (MD): AAZPA; 1987.
38. Cox C. Increase in the frequency of social interactions and the likelihood of reproduction among drills. In: AAZPA Regional Conference Proceedings. Bethesda (MD): AAZPA; 1987.
39. Rummel RJ. Aggression and the conflict helix. Understanding conflict and war: vol. 3: conflict in perspective. Beverly Hills (CA): Sage Publications; 1977.
40. Pryor K. Don't shoot the dog! The new art of teaching and training. United Kingdom: Ringpress Books; 2002.
41. Schapiro SJ. Effects of social manipulations and environmental enrichment on behavior and cell-mediated immune responses in rhesus macaques. J Pharmacol Biochem Behav 2002;73:271–8.
42. Desmond TJ, Laule GE. Use of positive reinforcement training in the management of species for reproduction. Zoo Biol 1984;13:471–7.
43. Forthman DL, Ogden JJ. The role of behavior analytic principles in zoo management: today and tomorrow. J Appl Behav Anal 1992;25:647–52.
44. Line SW, Clarke AD, Markowitz H. Plasma cortisol of female rhesus monkeys in response to acute restraint. Laboratory Primate Newsletter 1987;26:1–4.
45. Line SW, Morgan KN, Markowitz H, et al. Heart rate and activity of rhesus monkeys in response to routine events. Laboratory Primate Newsletter 1989;28:9–12.
46. Hediger H. Wild animals in captivity. London: Butterworth; 1950.
47. Laule G. The role of fear in abnormal behavior and animal welfare. In: Proceedings of the International conference on Environmental Enrichment. San Deigo (CA): Shape of Enrichment; 2005.
48. Clay AW, Bloomsmith MA, Marr MJ, et al. Habituation and desensitization as methods for reducing fearful behavior in singly housed rhesus macaques. Am J Primatol 2009;71:30–9.
49. Brain PF, Benton D. Multidisciplinary approach to aggression research. Amsterdam: Elsevier/North Holland Press; 1981.
50. Moyer KE. Kinds of aggression and their physiological basis. Commun Behav Biol A 1968;2:65–87.
51. Shepherdson DJ, Mellen JD, Hutchins M. Second nature: environmental enrichment for captive animals. Washington, DC: Smithsonian Institution; 1998.

Training Fish and Aquatic Invertebrates for Husbandry and Medical Behaviors

Allison L. Corwin, BS(Biology)

KEYWORDS

- Fish • Fishes • Aquatic invertebrates • Operant conditioning • Training • Learning
- Husbandry • Aquarium

KEY POINTS

- Outside of training animals for research purposes, very little peer-reviewed literature exists on training fishes and aquatic invertebrates.
- An animal's ability to learn is an essential component to training.
- The fundamentals of training fishes and invertebrates are similar to those of other animals.
- To develop an effective and useful training regime for fishes and aquatic invertebrates, the framework of the SPIDER method can be used: Setting goals, Planning, Implementing, Documenting, Evaluating, and Readjusting.
- Training a fish or aquatic invertebrate can provide early indication of health status prior to seeing physical signs of illness.

INTRODUCTION

Taking care of fishes and aquatic invertebrates has been an age-old tradition since the Roman Empire.[1] Throughout history it has progressed beyond just raising fish for food. It has developed into a well-established, personal hobby as well as a profession. Today there are more than 400 nonprofit and commercially affiliated professional aquariums around the world, and an estimated 151.1 million freshwater and 8.61 million saltwater fishes owned as personal pets in the United States alone.[2] This increasing popularity has led to an interest in advancing the quality of care and medical treatment of these species. Training fishes and aquatic invertebrates is one of the many ways that care can be improved.

Apart from training animals for research purposes, very little peer-reviewed literature exists on training fishes and aquatic invertebrates. However, over the past few years aquarists have started to report the ability to train these animals for husbandry

Animals, Science and the Environment, Disney's The Seas®, 2020 North Avenue of the Stars, Lake Buena Vista, FL 32830, USA
E-mail address: Allison.Corwin@disney.com

Vet Clin Exot Anim 15 (2012) 455–467
http://dx.doi.org/10.1016/j.cvex.2012.06.009
1094-9194/12/$ – see front matter © 2012 Elsevier Inc. All rights reserved.

and medical purposes in non–peer-reviewed journals, magazines, and conference proceedings. The goals of training fishes and aquatic invertebrates vary depending on the need of the animal, the trainer, and the facility. Training projects with fishes and invertebrates for husbandry and medical needs are usually centralized around at least one of the following goals: nutrition and dietary management, voluntary animal handling/capture techniques, and voluntary participation in medical procedures, leading to the overall aim of providing better animal care and enrichment to fishes and invertebrates in human care.

An animal's ability to learn is an essential component to training. Fishes and aquatic invertebrates are often perceived as evolutionary primitive species capable of only basic behaviors and instinctual responses; however, the more caretakers and researchers investigate these species, the more is learned about their complex behavioral repertoires and their extensive learning capabilities.

In an ever-changing aquatic environment, the ability to learn is critical to a fish's and invertebrate's livelihood. Since the 1800s experimentation in both wild and aquarium settings have demonstrated that fishes have similar learning capacities to those of birds and mammals.[3] For example, studies have shown that fishes can learn through observational, spatial, and aversion learning, enabling them to learn migration routes,[4] find food sources,[5] orient in their surroundings,[6] and avoid predators and unpalatable foods.[7]

The learning capabilities of aquatic invertebrates have been studied to a lesser extent with the exception of the class Cephalopoda, which includes animals such as octopus and cuttlefish. With no protective armament and short life spans, cephalopods benefit from the ability to learn to ensure their survival. Most experiments with cephalopods have demonstrated the learning potential of these animals through visual and tactile discrimination,[8] spatial learning using mazes in the laboratory and in the wild,[9,10] and avoidance learning.[11] Every species and individual animal may differ in their capabilities, but understanding that they can learn can lay the foundation for many useful training programs.

TRAINING FUNDAMENTALS

The fundamentals of training fishes and invertebrates are similar to those of other animals. A basic process of learning, such as classical conditioning, is often used in a research setting to test sensory abilities of fishes and invertebrates by using their natural reflexes in response to a learned association to a neutral stimulus. Operant conditioning is a type of learning process whereby the animal's voluntary behavior (or response) in the presence of a cue (or stimulus) is determined by its consequences, such as obtaining desired items/ events or avoiding aversives.[12] This learning process with an emphasis on positive reinforcement is typically the primary method used when teaching more complex behaviors, such as those needed for husbandry or medical behaviors. Positive reinforcement is often used to train an animal to target (touch some part of its body to another object), and is a useful training tool in aquatic environments.[12]

In most fish and aquatic invertebrate training, primary reinforcers (such as food), which serve a biological need of the animal, are used as the desired consequence in positive reinforcement training. Successful trainers find the correct dietary amount to achieve suitable nutrition as well as to maintain animal motivation. Secondary reinforcers can be used as well.

Secondary reinforcers are objects or events (stimuli) that through pairing with a primary reinforcer can themselves become reinforcing. These types of reinforcers can be used to help shape a desired behavior if food is no longer of interest or if the allotted amount of food has already been distributed.[12] A bridging stimulus is a secondary reinforcer that denotes a desired behavior before a reinforcer is delivered. Using a bridge is helpful in aquatic environments when the reinforcer may not be able to be offered immediately after the desired behavior is performed. Submerged clickers, generated underwater tones, body touching, and light signals are examples of bridges that can be used successfully in fishes and cephalopods.[13]

DEVELOPMENT OF TRAINING PLAN

To develop an effective and useful training regime for fishes and aquatic invertebrates, the framework of the SPIDER method can be used.[14] By following successive steps of Setting goals, Planning, Implementing, Documenting, Evaluating, and Readjusting (SPIDER), this method can provide a strategic approach to establishing training programs for fishes and aquatic invertebrates. In the initial planning, it is important to investigate the animal's natural and individual history, behavior, and sensory capabilities to understand how the animal learns and perceives the environment.

Natural History and Behavior

Because of the vast diversity of fishes and aquatic invertebrates, natural histories are expansive. Determining an animal's social structure (ie, solitary or social), common habitat (ie, pelagic or benthic), primary sensory modalities, activity pattern (ie, diurnal or nocturnal), diet choice (ie, herbivorous, omnivorous, or carnivorous), and food-consumption technique (ie, foragers or predators) can give directions in finding the correct training regime.

Individual histories can be just as vast, because every animal can differ in their environmental experiences and behavior. Examples include knowledge of the animal's origin (ie, wild caught or captive born), medical history, behavioral tendencies, and previous training history. Individual histories can give imperative insight into the animal's abilities and needs.[15]

Sensory

When developing a training plan, knowing how an animal perceives its environment can be very beneficial in understanding its behaviors and learning capabilities. Both physiologic and anatomic information is vast within the literature for many of these species, and a thorough literature search should be performed to help determine the specific sensory capabilities of fishes and invertebrates. These abilities can be different among aquatic animals, and some generalities are discussed here.

Studies have shown that most fishes have vision capabilities comparable with other vertebrates.[16] Fishes have highly developed eyes that allow for color vision in most bony fishes, and the ability to differentiate between color variation by contrasting light and dark colors in elasmobranchs.[16,17] Fishes have the capability to smell and taste chemical cues in the water through contact with chemoreceptors in their nares and mouths, and on their bodies. In sharks, olfaction capabilities are highly sensitive, being able to detect the presence of food as low as 100 parts per billion.[18] Fishes use their inner ears as well as their swim bladders, if present, to hear. Fishes can detect different frequencies centralized around lower pitches of 30 to 3000 Hz.[19] Because sharks do not have swim bladders, their hearing is slightly acute, responding to frequencies of 55 to 500 Hz.[18] Fishes also perceive their environment through a unique lateral line system consisting of rows of pores along the flank and head as well as free-standing sensory pores found on their bodies.[18] This system is used by fishes to detect information about low-frequency vibrations, water flow, and acceleration. Some fishes, such as cartilaginous fishes, catfish, and 2 species of African notopterids, have the ability to perceive natural electrical impulses called electroprecention.[19] These fishes use a passive ampullary form of electroreception to detect low electrical fields produced by muscle contractions and nerve impulses of prey buried under the substrate.[19,20] Sharks can detect voltage signals as low as 5 nV/cm.[21] Animals that use the active tuberous form of electroreception, such as electric eels, have specialize electric organs that can produce an electric field around them to gather information about their surroundings as well as use their ability to stun prey, discourage predators, and communicate with each other.[19,22]

Aquatic invertebrates' vision capabilities range from bivalves, which only have light photoreceptor cells that detect shadows and movement, to cephalopods, which have sophisticated eyesight that cannot discriminate amongst colors but are capable of seeing polarized light.[23] Most species of aquatic invertebrates smell or taste the water by using chemoreceptors on their tentacles or arms, or located around their siphons. This method enables them to find prey and detect other chemical stimulants in the water, such as turbidity.[24] In most aquatic invertebrates, an analog of the fish's inner ear called the statocyst is present. Although hearing is not its function, this enables invertebrates to detect body position in relation to gravity as well as to detect acceleration in different directions, as found in crabs.[23,24] In most aquatic invertebrates, mechanoreceptors can be found dispersed over the body, as well as in concentrated areas that are specifically used for sensory perception. In the case of squid, epidermal lines of hair cells on the head and arms can detect directionality of signals from their prey, predators, or conspecifics.[18,23] Knowing how the particular animal being trained perceives its environment is critical, and can be helpful in determining the approaches used to train it.

OBJECTIVES

Because of the extent of their innate capabilities, sensory competencies, and learning capacity, aquarists and veterinarians can use this information about fishes and aquatic invertebrates to develop training programs that aid in daily husbandry and medical needs of these animals in human care, including training for dietary management, capture techniques, and medical procedures.

Dietary Management

Diet regulation is critical in maintaining good health of fishes and aquatic invertebrates. Sometimes supplying the correct, balanced diet is not enough. Delivery is often the challenge. Uncontrolled feedings can often lead to obesity or anorexia, and sometimes injury caused by competing for food. By implementing a training regime, aquarists can deliver foods to animals with special needs and cater to their different feeding strategies. Training also can minimize or eliminate interspecies and intraspecies competition for food by controlling the delivery in an organized fashion, especially when many animals are involved. Training can also enable aquarists to collect individual consumption information to determine daily dietary requirements of specific animals, which could include vitamin supplementation.

Overeating

Overeating can lead to many medical issues. In every aquarium, there always seems to be at least one animal that outcompetes the others for food. This situation often leads to obesity, which can be directly related to other health issues. Training these individuals can help regulate the overeater's diet as well as help other animals in the exhibit obtain the proper nutrition.

An example of this is found in a saltwater fish, the cobia (*Rachycentron canadum*). These fish are a widely cultured species primarily used in the food industry, but are often found in aquariums because of their unique look, large size, and active swim pattern. Historically at Disney's The Seas, cobia tend to have weight issues owing to overeating in the mixed species environment, leading to exophthalmia caused by large fat deposits behind their eyes. To restrict a specific individual's diet, the cobia at The Seas was trained to relocate to a particular location in the exhibit to prevent it from overeating during the general population feed. In one particular case, an animal was trained to respond and target on a white polyvinylchloride (PVC) "T," 2 cm in diameter, submerged about 30 cm under the water's surface. When the animal saw this cue in conjunction with an auditory/mechanoreceptive cue of splashing the water's surface, it approached the location and repeatedly stationed at the PVC target for 1 to 5 small pieces of food until its allotted amount was delivered (**Fig. 1**). Care was taken to evenly distribute the food at a rate to encourage the animal to stay in this location while the main population feed occurred 6 m away. Location and time of day of the training was kept consistent in accordance with the spatial[5] and temporal learning capabilities of fishes.[25] By training this animal to target and station, aquarists were able to provide the cobia with the properly reduced diet it needed, as well as nutritional supplementation.[26]

Slow or less aggressive eaters
Some animals are slow and less assertive eaters, whether it is due to their natural history or as a result of aggressive behavior from other animals during feeding times. To ensure they receive their diet, training can be useful to redirect them to a more secure area to feed.

Slow-moving echinoderms have a difficult time competing for food when housed with active teleosts. A Bahamian seastar *(Oreaster reticulates)* at Disney's The Seas was trained to eat at the surface of a tank to minimize food stealing from fish in the exhibit and offer the water's surface as another form of protection. Initially, training started by picking up the seastar and moving it to the desired location near the surface of the tank to be fed. After about a week, the seastar started spending more time near the top of the tank and was fed by aquarists when they observed this behavior. An added bonus of the training was that the sides of the tank were clear acrylic, which

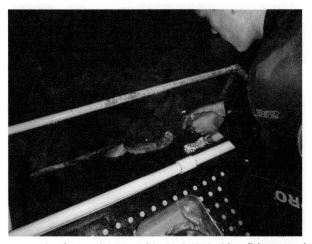

Fig. 1. Cobia target trained to station at a white PVC "T" inside a fish pen to deliver diet and nutritional supplementation at Disney's The Seas.

allows visitors to see how the seastar eats (John Dickson, Sr Aquarist, Disney's The Seas, Lake Buena Vista, FL, personal communication, February 2012).

Aggressive behavior

Aggressive behavior is often observed when fishes compete over territory, mates, status, and food. With regard to food, training has helped reduce aggressive behavior during feeding sessions, alleviating injuries and allowing all animals to acquire the appropriate amounts of food.

Such was the case for one exhibit at Disney's The Seas, which contained 3 different species of eels: 6 snowflake morays (*Echidna nebulosa*), 4 leopard snake eels (*Myrichthys pardalis*), and 2 zebra morays (*Gymnomuraena zebra*). The 12 eels were all housed together in a 1136-L display exhibit. During feeding times, the snowflake eels showed aggressive behavior and continuously stole food from the other eels. This aggression resulted in irregular diets and occasional trauma caused by bites. In response to this problem, aquarists developed a training plan specifically for the snowflake eels, to make the feed more organized and address aggressive behavior. Knowing eels naturally occupy crevices or holes in the reef, aquarists used this tendency and constructed a feeding apparatus that contained 4 clear, 5.08-cm diameter, PVC pipes connected parallel to each other, and hung it vertically in the tank (**Fig. 2**). After conditioning the eels to eat from a feeding stick, they were trained to follow the stick with food into the pipes and feed near the surface of the water. Even if the some of the eels did not participate in the pipe training, the larger eels, which were much more food motivated, were distracted enough in the pipes for aquarists to be able to train the smaller snowflake eels to learn the behavior as well. It also allowed aquarists to document food intake for each eel and provided an educational experience for visitors of the facility (John Dickson, Sr Aquarist, Disney's The Seas, Lake Buena Vista, FL, personal communication, February 2012).

Target training has also been successfully used to reduce aggressive behavior, such as chasing and biting, in shark species. Aquarists at the Rotterdam Zoo in the Netherlands divided their pelagic shark species into 2 groups: (1) 4 blacknose sharks (*Carcharhinus acronotus*), and (2) 3 sandbar sharks (*Carcharhinus plumbeus*) and 2 blacktip sharks (*Carcharhinus limbatus*). By training each group to a specific visual

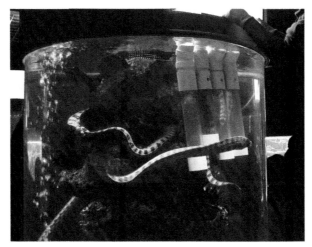

Fig. 2. Snowflake eels trained to swim into a PVC pipe apparatus to feed at Disney's The Seas.

target at 2 locations of a multispecies exhibit, aquarists noted an 80% reduction in the behavior problems that occurred during feedings.[27]

Because of their size and strength, some animals can be difficult if not dangerous for aquarists to feed. Target training an animal can reduce aggressive behavior toward the feeder and lead to an organized, safer feed. At Disney's The Seas, spotted eagle rays (*Aetobatus narinari*) were hand-fed by scuba divers in a large 8.2-m deep aquarium. For educational purposes, the spotted eagle rays were trained to come close to the visitor-viewing windows to feed. Initially, the aquarists carried the rays' food in inconsistent locations, such as in their hands, wetsuits, and/or dive-gear pockets. When the animal approached, food was delivered. The rays quickly learned where the food was located and started biting at the diver's gear, bumping off masks and pulling out regulator hoses if food was not delivered quickly enough. To reduce aggressive behaviors, aquarists started associating a visual target (10.16-cm diameter white PVC elbow with a nylon handle) with food delivery, eventually requiring the rays to touch their rostrum to the target in a controlled, horizontal position to earn reinforcers. This training significantly decreased the aggressive behavior of the stingrays and provided a more controlled, safer feed.[28]

Managing large populations

Many facilities have large groups of animals that require dietary management. The delivery of food must be relatively rapid and in an organized fashion. At a stingray interaction program in the Bahamas, more than 60 southern stingrays (*Dasyatis americana*) were trained to swim up a ramp and around a floating platform submerged approximately 30.5 cm under water. While the animals were in the floating station, they were trained to stop over a black, flat, polyethylene target to be hand-fed by both aquarists and visitors. During this time, animals were inspected physically for appropriate body condition. Participation rate in feeding sessions was documented, keeping track of which animals were eating routinely (Erin Rombough, Disney's Aquarist, Castaway Cay, the Bahamas, personal communication, February 2012).[29]

Tank size

Irregularly shaped or deep tanks can make it challenging to provide some animals with proper nutrition. If diving to feed the fish or aquatic invertebrate is not possible, training benthic animals to come to the surface for easier feeding is sometimes required. Many species of sharks have been trained to feed at the surface of deep exhibits in response to a physical target, feeding-platform locations, or a bright light that can penetrate deep into the water during early morning hours when light levels are low and animals are most active (Larry Rutherford, Disney's Sr Aquarist, Lake Buena Vista, FL, personal communication, February 2012).[13] If possible, training an animal in a smaller, shallower holding tank before relocating it to a deeper and bigger exhibit can build the strength of the training and can often make the transfer of the behavior to the bigger exhibit more successful. Incorporating sensory cues of olfaction (chumming the water), auditory (tapping on the plastic target with the metal feeding tongs), and mechanoreception (splashing the water's surface) with the desired target can also increase the response time of the animal.

Voluntary Capture Techniques

Catching an aquatic animal can prove difficult and stressful for both the animals and the caretakers. Incorporating capture devices, such as nets, fish pens, and stretchers, into daily feeding regimes desensitizes the animals to these devices. Training an animal to swim through or stop inside a capture device during routine sessions enables aquarists to use them when needed while inducing less stress in the animal.

In coordination with the diet-regulation training of the cobia from the previous example, a capture plan was also devised because of the fish's size and strength. A pen (91.4 × 121.9 × 55.9 cm) made out of 2.54-cm PVC pipe and black netting was added under the surface platform where the fish was trained to target (see **Fig. 1**). To be reinforced, the animal had to swim into the front open panel of the pen to the target. The pen was large enough that the cobia was able to swim into and out of the pen throughout the session. When it was time to capture the animal for physical examination or to transfer it into another exhibit, the animal entered the pen and approached the target as usual. The open side of the pen was then closed, containing the animal for easier capture.[26]

Stingrays are common in many public aquariums and require routine captures for annual examinations. Because this requires multiple handlings, aquarists train behaviors to minimize stress during captures. At The Georgia Aquarium, manta rays (*Manta birostris*), which can reach maximum disk widths of 9 m and weigh up to 1350 kg, were trained daily to follow colored ladles of food over submerged, large stretchers. Through successive approximations, the stretchers were gradually positioned so that the exit water depth was shallower than the entrance depth. When the animal needed to be captured for routine physicals or medical treatments, the exit depth was raised so that the manta ray partially beached itself when it swam through, containing it in a shallower pool of water inside the stretcher.[30]

Animals that are more difficult to handle, such as sharks, can be trained to swim into smaller tanks, such as a holding or medical pool, to eat, aiding in easier and safer captures. A zebra shark (*Stegostoma fasciatum*) at Disney's The Seas was trained to follow a target pole (2.54-cm diameter white PVC "T" glued on top of a 1.5-m long, 2.54-cm diameter PVC pipe) into a smaller enclosure at the surface of an 8.2-m deep exhibit to eat. When needed, this training allowed aquarists to place a stretcher on the bottom of the crate and easily lift it up and around the animal when it was positioned over it. This maneuver made it easier to catch the shark in a smaller space in comparison with trying to catch it in a 21.5-million-liter exhibit.

In aquaculture, fishes can be trained to aid harvesting techniques. By pairing an acoustic cue with food, fishes were trained to come into a small location of a larger aquaponics pond to be fed daily and then eventually harvested in that location.[31]

Voluntary Participation in Medical Procedures

Training an animal to voluntarily participate in a medical procedure can be a much more efficient way to obtain medical diagnostics or therapeutics. Delivering medicated food, obtaining basic information such as skin scrapes and morphometrics, stationing animals for ultrasound examination, or even just getting close enough to them in the water can often be done voluntarily by the animal and without anesthesia. This method greatly reduces the stress on the animal and may prevent the need for more invasive procedures.

Delivering oral medication

Routine delivery of medication is often needed to treat a diagnosed illness or infection in an animal. If medication can be delivered orally and in a controlled manner, the stress of capturing the animal and handling it can be eliminated if the animal is trained to be hand fed. Aquarists at the Monterey Bay Aquarium consistently experience trematode infestations on their California bat rays (*Myliobatis californica*). By training the rays to hand feed from a scuba diver using a visual target (white circular disk with a black "X") and consistent feeding location in their large 1.26-million-liter system, aquarists were able to successfully deliver oral droncit/biltricide (praziquantel) to each individual to treat the trematode infestation.[32]

Skin scrapes and morphometrics

Skin scrapes of a fish or invertebrate are often a part of a routine examination, and results can be clear indicators of parasitic infestation. Training a fish to be held partially out of the water for a short period of time or to remain stationary long enough underwater to get a successful scrape can be beneficial and easily done.

Using food as a reinforcer, an aquarist from New England Aquarium trained a lumpfish (*Cyclopterus lumpus*) to voluntarily swim into her hand, remain calm when lifted partially out of the water, and allow the scraping of its flank with a coverslip of a microscope slide as a part of its physical examination.[33]

On a larger scale, goliath groupers (*Epinephelus itajara*) at Disney's The Seas were trained to be approached by divers to not only hand feed and regulate diet[34] but to also station for longer periods of time to gather basic medical information. Because goliath groupers are strong and fast, catching them can be difficult and potentially harmful to both the animal and the capturer. Training groupers to hand feed has been shown to develop a positive association between the caretaker and fish, allowing aquarists to routinely get close to the animal without creating a fear response.

Besides primary reinforcers, such as food, secondary reinforcers have also been used successfully in training goliath groupers. At Disney's The Seas, aquarists found that trickling crushed scallop shell over the bodies and gills of the groupers ("shelling") provided desired tactile stimulation that not only captured the attention of the goliath groupers but also the black and red groupers, *Mycteroperca bonaci* and *Epinephelus morio*, respectively. By pairing "shelling" with a visual target (30.5-cm pink, hexagonal acrylic sheet with a handle), aquarists easily trained goliath groupers to follow a target and to station for longer periods of time. This method enabled divers to lead the animals into a capture device such as a crate, where they obtained girth and length measurements, and were able to routinely observe gills and eyes, and perform skin scrapes under water (**Fig. 3**). The participation rate of this training using secondary reinforcers has sometimes proved to be more successful than using food reinforcers throughout the year, because of the groupers' fluctuating appetites.[26]

Sharks can also be trained to voluntarily participate in medical procedures. Zebra sharks, *Stegostoma fasciatum*, at Pittsburgh Zoo and PPG Aquarium were target trained and desensitized to tactile stimulation to provide controlled feedings and

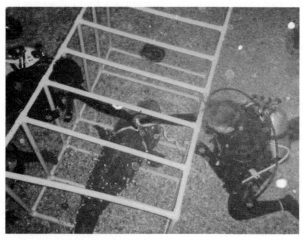

Fig. 3. Goliath grouper target training at Disney's The Seas to assist in morphometric measurements and mock-crate desensitization.

facilitate medical procedures. Through successive approximations and positive reinforcement, the initial target training of this benthic species to eat at the surface quickly developed into desensitizing the animals to accept touch. By pairing the strong targeting behavior with the trainer's light touch and reinforcers, the animals quickly became desensitized to tactile pressure. Through shaping with successive approximations, the animals accepted the gradual increase of touch until aquarists were able to hold the animals in place for a period of time to be able to measure their total length and to give intramuscular injections. Animals were also inverted for ventral inspections and to obtain voluntary blood samples. The zebra sharks were also desensitized to being lifted out of the water for a short period of time to obtain weights.[35]

Invertebrates, such as the giant Pacific octopus (GPO), *Enteroctopus dofleini*, can be trained to voluntarily participate in medical procedures. Many caretakers of the GPO develop enrichment programs as well as train them to assist in routine husbandry needs associated with medical examinations, such as tactile desensitization and voluntary weights. By using shaping with successive approximations, a GPO at Pittsburgh Zoo and PPG Aquarium was trained to approach the top of the tank when the trainer slapped on the water's surface. A tactile cue of gently tugging on the animal's arm 2 times and placing the juice of its food (squid) on the wall of the tank encouraged the GPO to eventually travel out of the tank and into a plastic container to be weighed. After obtaining the weight, the animal crawled back into its exhibit and was reinforced with food and tactile stimulation.[36]

Ultrasound

Training an animal to station voluntarily for long periods of time or for successive trials can be helpful when ultrasound is needed. A target can be used to teach an animal to station. Teaching the animal to hold position on the station for long duration can be done by using a bridging stimulus and food reinforcers. Desensitizing the animal through repeated exposure to other people in or around the water as well as introducing controlled touch on their dorsal surfaces during stationing can be helpful. By using this technique, aquarists and veterinarians can work together to monitor pregnant animals, such as stingrays, without having to capture the animal or use anesthesia. Capture can be stressful, and has caused premature birthing and loss of the pups. Aquarists at Parque Nizuc, Cancun, Mexico trained benthic elasmobrachs, such as nurse sharks (*Ginglymostoma cirratum*), southern stingrays (*Dasyatis americana*), and chupare stingrays (*Dasyatis schmardae*), to lie on top of PVC tables submerged approximately 35 cm below the surface for voluntary ultrasound and other medical procedures.[29] Pelagic stingrays, such as the spotted eagle ray (*Aetobatus narinari*), have also been trained for voluntary ultrasound with a slight difference in the target. Unlike benthic species of stingrays, pelagic stingrays are constantly swimming. Staying stationary is slightly harder to train but can be achieved by providing a stable target for the animal's rostrum.[26] By allowing the animal to apply pressure to the stable target in conjunction with moving its wings slightly, the animal can remain stationary for short periods of time (**Fig. 4**) (Tanya Kamerman, Aquarist, Disney's The Seas, Lake Buena Vista, FL, personal communication, February 2012).

Behavioral Indicators of Health

Training a fish or aquatic invertebrate can provide an early indication of health status before seeing physical signs of illness. Every training session can teach caretakers more about the animals on an individual level, providing baseline behavioral information that can be used as a comparison at later times. For example, if an animal is always consistent in training participation, inconsistencies can alert the caretaker

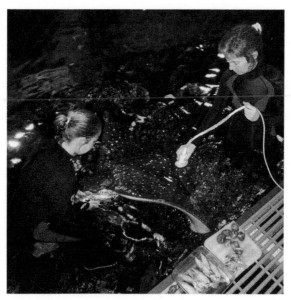

Fig. 4. Spotted eagle ray trained to remain stationary on a target while a veterinary ultra-sounds at Disney's The Seas.

about a potential illness or injury. Earlier alerts can increase the odds of treating the problem, as was the case for the cobia from the previous examples.

After eating reliably for months, the cobia started to reduce its diet by spitting out items and refusing food. Because of the behavioral patterns established in training, aquarists knew this change in feeding pattern was unusual for this individual and were on alert. By day 3, the animal started showing signs of irregular swimming, and veterinarians were notified. On day 4, the animal continued to participate in training sessions and perform behaviors even though it was not eating, which allowed aquarists to use the trained capture technique and quickly move the animal to a medical tank. On medical examination, the fish showed signs of infection and received extensive medical treatment. After about a month, the target was reintroduced into the holding tank in attempt to get the fish to feed on its own. The animal responded well and despite the change of environment and medical setbacks, the cobia approached the target and started eating again.

SUMMARY

Training can be helpful in many aspects of a captive animal's life, as observed in the cobia and other examples in this article. Because fishes and invertebrates have the capacity to learn, caretakers can use this ability to provide an increased level of care through training, thus facilitating overall health, enrichment, and animal welfare in captive aquatic environments.

REFERENCES

1. Beltrame C, Gaddi D, Parizzi S. A presumed hydraulic apparatus for the transport of live fish, found on the roman wreck at Grado, Italy. Int J Nautical Archaeology 2011;40:274–82.

2. American Pet Products Manufacturer Association. National pet owners survey 2011-2012. Available at: http://www.americanpetproducts.org/press_industrytrends.asp. Accessed February 1, 2012.
3. Kieffer JD, Colgan PW. The role of learning in fish behavior. Rev Fish Biol Fish 1992;2:125–43.
4. Helfman GS, Schultz ET. Social transmission of behavioural traditions in a coral reef fish. Anim Behav 1984;32:379–84.
5. Dill LM. Adaptive flexibility in the foraging behavior of fishes. Can J Fish Aquat Sci 1983;40(4):398–408.
6. Dodson JJ. The nature and role of learning in orientation and migratory behaviour of fishes. Environ Biol Fish 1998;23:161–82.
7. Kruse KC, Stone BM. Largemouth bass (Micropterus salmoides) learn to avoid feeding on toad (Bufo) tadpoles. Anim Behav 1984;32:1035–9.
8. Messenger JB. Learning in the cuttlefish, Sepia. Anim Behav 1973;21(4):801–26.
9. Karson MA, Boal JG, Hanlon RT. Experimental evidence for spatial learning in cuttlefish (Sepia officinalis). J Comp Psychol 2003;117(2):149–55.
10. Boal JG, Dunham AW, Williams KT, et al. Experimental evidence for spatial learning in octopuses (Octopus bimaculoides). J Comp Psychol 2000;114(3):246–52.
11. Darmaillacq AS, Dickel L, Chichery MP, et al. Rapid taste aversion learning in adult cuttlefish, Sepia officinalis. Anim Behav 2004;68(6):1291–8.
12. Ramirez K. Animal training: successful management through positive reinforcement. Chicago: John G. Shedd Aquarium; 1999.
13. Sabalones J, Walters H, Bohorquez CA. Learning and behavioral enrichment in elasmobranchs. In: Smith M, Warmolts D, Thoney D, et al, editors. Elasmobranch husbandry manual: captive care of sharks, rays, and their relatives. Columbus (OH): Biological Survey, Inc; 2004. p. 169–82.
14. Mellen J, Sevenich MacPhee M. Animal training framework. 2002. Disney's Animal Kingdom® Theme Park. Available at: www.animaltraining.org. Accessed March 1, 2012.
15. Disney's Animal Science and Environment, Behavioral Husbandry Team. Disney's animal programs training philosophy and expectations. Available at: http://www.animaltraining.org/training%20philosophy.htm. Accessed February 1, 2012.
16. Helfman GS. The diversity of fishes: biology, evolution, and ecology. 2nd edition. Chichester (United Kingdom): Blackwell; 2009. p. 84–7.
17. Greenberg J, Greenberg I. Sharks and other dangerous sea creatures. Miami (FL): Seahawk Press; 1981. p. 62.
18. Reinert RE. Fish physiology. In: Gratzek JB, Matthews JR, editors. Aquariology, master volume. Morris Plains (NJ): Tetra Press; 1992. p. 161–86.
19. Reebs S. Fish behavior in the aquarium and in the wild. Ithaca (NY): Cornell University Press; 2001. p. 26.
20. Coplin SP, Whitehead D. The functional roles of passive electroreception in non-electric fishes. Anim Biol 2004;54(1):1–25.
21. Kalmijn AJ. Electric and magnetic field detection in elasmobranch fishes. Science 1982;218:916–8.
22. Albert JS, Crampton WG. Electroreception and electrogenesis. In: Lutz PL, editor. The physiology of fishes. Boca Raton (FL): CRC Press; 2006. p. 429–70.
23. Ruppert EE, Fox RS, Barnes RD. Mollusca. In: Invertebrate zoology. 7th edition. Philadelphia: Brooks/Cole; 2004. p. 283–412.
24. Ruppert EE, Fox RS, Barnes RD. Crustacea. In: Invertebrate zoology. 7th edition. Philadelphia: Brooks/Cole; 2004. p. 605–701.

25. Boujard T, Leatherland JF. Circadian rhythms and feeding time in fishes. Environ Biol Fish 1992;35:109–31.
26. Davis LM. Training and enrichment in aquariums—not just for dolphins anymore. NAVC Conference Proceedings (North American Veterinary Conference). Orlando (FL): Gaylord Palms; 2010.
27. Laterveer M. Changing the feeding regime in a multi-species open-ocean tank by means of target training pelagic sharks. Drum and Croaker. 2006. Available at: http://www.columbuszoo.org/drumcroaker/pdf/2006.pdf. Accessed February 1, 2012.
28. Muraco HS, Stamper MA. Training spotted eagle rays (*Aetobatus narinari* (Euphrasen)) to decrease aggressive behaviors towards divers. J Aquariculture Aquat Sci 2003;8(4):88–98.
29. Wilson A, Davis J. A mouse among rays! Drum and Croaker. 2008. Available at: http://www.columbuszoo.org/drumcroaker/pdf/2008.pdf. Accessed February 1, 2012.
30. Christen DR, Schreiber CM. Stretcher training of a giant manta (*Manta birostris*) to facilitate physical examinations. Soundings 2010;35(2):12–5.
31. Levin LE, Levin AF. Conditioning as an aid to fish harvest. Aquacult Eng 1994; 13(3):201–10.
32. Leward K. Underwater training, feeding and medication for California Bat Rays, *Myliobatis californica* in large community exhibits. Drum & Croaker. 2006. Available at: http://www.columbuszoo.org/drumcroaker/pdf/2006.pdf. Accessed February 1, 2012.
33. New England Aquarium. Lumpfish trained to get skin scrape. 2009. Available at: www.youtube.com/watch?v=9KvrLug6NjA. Accessed February 1, 2012.
34. Ratte ME, Kittell MM. Monitoring feed amounts in goliath groupers (*Epinephelus itajara*) using behavioral conditioning in a large mixed species exhibit. Zoo Biol 2008;27(5):414–9.
35. Snowden R. Target training and tactile conditioning of two zebra sharks, *Stegostoma fasciatum*. Drum and Croaker. 2008. Available at: http://www.columbuszoo.org/drumcroaker/pdf/2008.pdf. Accessed February 1, 2012.
36. Moffatt J. The training of a male giant Pacific octopus, *Enteroctopus dofleini* to assess health and weight. Drum and Croaker. 2007. Available at: http://www.columbuszoo.org/drumcroaker/pdf/2007.pdf. Accessed February 1, 2012.

Small Mammal Training in the Veterinary Practice

Susan A. Brown, DVM

KEYWORDS

- Positive reinforcement • Training • Veterinary • Rabbit • Rodent • Ferret

KEY POINTS

- In the past, veterinary intervention involving small mammals often resulted in creating a fearful patient as well as damaging the bond the patient may have had with the client.
- Desensitization, counterconditioning, and positive reinforcement training are all excellent strategies to reduce fear in small mammal patients both in and outside of the veterinary practice.
- Clients can use positive reinforcement to train a number of simple health care behaviors at home, creating a patient that will willingly participate in veterinary interventions.
- Veterinary staff members have many opportunities during an office visit to positively impact a small mammal patient and build a bond of trust with both the patient and the client.

 Videos of training of rats, rabbits, and guinea pigs accompany this article at http://www.vetexotic.theclinics.com/

INTRODUCTION

Veterinarians take an oath that includes the statement "I will… use my scientific knowledge and skills for … the prevention and relief of animal suffering." This has been at the heart of veterinary practice for decades even as veterinarians were not always aware of additional suffering inadvertently caused by their intervention. It was the lesser of two evils to cure the disease that might have killed, even though the patient may have been left in a state of fear when exposed to the veterinary staff and the client who administered the care. Many a trusting relationship between caregiver and companion animal has suffered serious and sometimes permanent damage in the aftermath of veterinary intervention.[1] Animals restrained overzealously and forced to endure aversive experiences can also be dangerous to the handler as they struggle to escape.[1] Small mammal patients often run frantically around their cages before being forcefully and quickly grabbed, bringing all 4 feet off the ground in order to be

PO Box 431, North Aurora, IL 60542, USA
E-mail address: behaviorconnection@earthlink.net

Vet Clin Exot Anim 15 (2012) 469–485
http://dx.doi.org/10.1016/j.cvex.2012.06.007   **vetexotic.theclinics.com**

examined. The "chase-grab-lift" scenario mimics a life-threatening predatory chase-and-capture situation. This stressful event might occur once or twice a day if the animal has to be treated for a disorder.

Over the past 20 years, increasing numbers of zoological parks and laboratories have successfully used positive reinforcement training to teach many species of animals to choose to cooperate in their own health care. The welfare of the animals is improved because heavy-handed restraint is eliminated, fear responses decrease significantly, the physiological changes of stress are reduced and the animals expand their repertoire of behaviors resulting in behavioral enrichment.[2–9] It has become popular in recent years to teach health care behaviors to cats, dogs, and parrots. Dog and cat trainers are conducting classes in veterinary clinics where puppies and kittens and their caregivers have positively reinforcing experiences with veterinary staff and the clinic environment. Parrots are also being trained using positive reinforcement to tolerate veterinary examinations and treatments.[10] This exciting movement is creating a new generation of companion animals that come to the veterinarian experienced, confident, and willing to cooperate in routine health care activities. This can be done with exotic small mammal patients as well.

The set of behaviors referred to in this chapter as "health care behaviors" may also be referred to as husbandry behaviors and/or medical behaviors. Health care behaviors include any behaviors performed by an animal that allows it to participate willingly in grooming, transportation, examination, medicating (topical, oral, or parenteral), and common diagnostic procedures. **Box 1** lists some common health care behaviors that are valuable to train. Once a behavior is trained, the key to the animal's success performing the behavior is a rich history of positive reinforcement built through many repetitions under nonaversive situations so that the animal predicts a positive valuable outcome each time. On the occasions when the procedure may be aversive, such as a bitter instead of palatable oral medication, the animal has such a dense history of

---

Box 1
Health care behaviors to train

- *Recall*: Approaching when called.
- *Crating*: Going into and coming out of a carrier and being moved in a carrier.
- *Being picked up and carried*: Or stepping onto an open hand.
- *Toweling*: Being able to be lightly restrained with a towel.
- *Examining*: Being able to apply pressure to and move various parts of the body.
- *Targeting*: Touching a body part to a target. This can be used for positioning or creating movement such as:
  - Getting onto and off of a scale
  - Staying in one area of the cage while it is cleaned (stationing)
  - Standing still while being treated/examined
  - Coming out of a cage
  - Standing in a clear box to be examined
- Oral, ear, and eye medicating
- Nail trimming
- Fur brushing

positive reinforcement it develops "behavioral resiliency" and bounces back more easily from the aversive experience, willing to trust the trainer (veterinary staff or caregiver) again relatively quickly.[11]

There are 2 main locations where health care behaviors in companion small mammals are trained: in the animal's home environment with the caregiver as the trainer and in the veterinary practice with the staff as trainers. The behavior principles used are the same in both situations and each place of training is equally valuable (**Box 2**).

SOURCES FOR INFORMATION ON TRAINING ANIMALS

There are many resources on training animals including texts, Web sites, specialty groups, videos, and workshops from which to choose. The veterinarian should consider finding a local veterinary behaviorist or animal trainer who uses positive reinforcement training strategies with either domestic or zoo animals. These individuals can assist in developing instructional materials for clients of exotic small mammals and can help train staff. See **Box 3** for a list of resources to get started including a list of behavior associations that are sources for trainers or behaviorists (see Videos 1–6 online at www.vetexotic.theclinics.com).

FIRST LEARN THE SIGNS OF FEAR

It is difficult to train new behaviors if the animal does not show behaviors indicative of comfort around the trainer. Veterinarians and caregivers wishing to interact effectively with animals must learn the body language related to discomfort, most notably fear and anxiety, a group of behaviors referred to hereafter in this article with the label fear behavior(s). When encountering a potentially threatening situation, an animal will present behaviors indicative of anxiety or fear as it works out how to handle the situation. Three common responses to a potential threat to safety in small mammals include freeze behavior, aggressive behavior, or fleeing behavior. An animal may exhibit 1 or more of these responses during a stressful experience and may switch rapidly between all 3 based on what is most effective at the moment.

In the author's experience, most small mammals presented at the veterinary practice will choose freeze behavior first. They often respond with sudden stillness accompanied by tension in body posture with wide-open, unblinking eyes. Freezing is a way of not being seen by a predator. Fleeing is usually the next choice. If flight is not an option, for instance for a caged animal that has no escape route, then the animal

---

Box 2
Benefits of training health care behaviors in exotic small mammals

- Creates a patient that willingly participates in health care procedures significantly reducing stress on the patient, the veterinary staff and the caregiver.
- Reduces patient aggressive behavior toward the veterinary staff or caregiver.[1]
- Preempts the need for heavy-handed or chemical restraint.
- Increases behavioral resiliency when it is necessary to expose the animal to an aversive experience. They "bounce back" more easily.[11]
- Builds a relationship of trust between caregiver and animal reducing the animal's anxiety and fear in its daily life.
- Creates empowering problem solving opportunities for the animal resulting in behavioral enrichment and an increase in the animal's behavioral repertoire.

Box 3
Behavior and training resources

Behavior Associations

- American Veterinary Society of Animal Behavior (AVSAB): www.avsabonline.org
- International Association of Animal Behavior Consultants (IAABC): www.iaabc.org
- Animal Behavior Management Alliance (ABMA): www.theabma.org
- Animal Behavior Society: www.animalbehaviorsociety.org

Exotic Animal Behavior/Training Texts and Videos

- *Exotic Pet Behavior: Birds, Reptiles, and Small Mammals.* Bradley Bays T, Lightfoot T, Mayer J. Saunders Elsevier 2006.
- *Behavior of Exotic Pets.* Tynes V ed. Wiley Blackwell 2010.
- *The Complete Guide to Rat Training.* Ducommun D. T.F.H. Publications 2008.
- *Getting Started: Clicking with your Rabbit.* Orr J, Lewin T. Sunshine Books, Inc 2006.
- *Bunny Training 101* (Video). Heidenreich B. 2011. www.bunnytraining.com

Websites

- www.behaviorworks.org: Dr Susan Friedman's website. Includes a large number of articles on principles of behavior and information on the course for animal professionals on applied behavior analysis called *Living and Learning with Animals.*
- www.drsophiayin.com: Sophia Yin, DVM's website. Although the focus is on dogs and cats, there are many valuable articles on the principles of behavior and training.
- www.clickertraining.com: Karen Pryor's website on all aspects of positive reinforcement using a clicker as a bridging stimulus or event marker covering a variety of species including small mammals.
- www.bunnytraining.com: Barbara Heidenreich's website about training rabbits.
- www.clickerbunny.com: Website devoted to clicker training in rabbits.
- www.kenramireztraining.com: Ken Ramirez's website including courses on learning about animal training.
- www.legacycanine.com: Terry Ryan's website with information on learning positive reinforcement training through Chicken Camps.

---

may resort to "fighting" or aggressive behavior. In the author's experience the majority of small mammals do not resort to aggressive behavior as their first defense. Therefore, the veterinary staff or client needs to learn early signs of fear or discomfort in order to respond appropriately to reduce the animal's discomfort. Animals that do present aggressive behaviors immediately have often learned in their home environment or in the veterinary environment that freezing and fleeing did not work to remove the aversive (the human) and fighting (biting, scratching, lunging) was reinforced as is the most effective strategy. Each time an aggressive behavior removes an aversive stimulus, the behavior is reinforced thus teaching the animal to repeat the aggressive behavior. Veterinarians should avoid becoming part of this aggressive behavior reinforcement cycle. Aggressive behavior can usually be avoided by not pressuring the animal to resort to this strategy. **Box 4** provides common fear behaviors in small mammals. As the caregiver and veterinary staff's observational skills improve, more subtle signs of anxiety or fear will be seen allowing earlier intervention in avoiding a flight or fight response.

Box 4
Common fear behaviors in rabbits, ferrets, and rodents

Rabbits

- Eyes wide open and unblinking, eyes bulging slightly
- Ears forward at first and then laid back against body (this is more difficult to observe in lop eared rabbits)
- Body still, body flattened to the ground
- Body stiff and weight in back legs
- Lunging with head and front feet, foot thumping, growling, grunting, biting

Ferrets[12]

- Piloerection on tail and sometimes body
- Hissing, huffing, screaming, anal gland expression
- Arched back, lunging, biting, backing up with mouth open (this can also be observed in play behavior)

Guinea Pig[13]

- Eyes wide, lowered head and ears, head stretched forward
- Shiver, freeze, stiffening of front legs, standing tall, feigning death
- Repeated nudging of cage bedding, constant digging

Rats

- High pitched squeal, low pitched squeak, hissing, teeth chattering
- Standing on hind legs, slapping tail, revealing lower teeth, lunging with mouth open, biting

Hamsters[14]

- Body stiffness, stand upright, flatten to the ground, washing face continuously
- Flip onto back with mouth open, defecating and urinating
- Screaming, tooth clicking, lunging and biting

Chinchillas

- Stiff body with weight in hind legs, ears forward, standing upright
- Teeth chattering, barking, screaming, grunting, whistling
- Urine spraying, lunging, biting

DESENSITIZATION

Desensitization is a behavior change strategy that gradually exposes an animal to an aversive stimulus in small enough increments so as not to elicit a strong fear reaction. The animal learns to relax over time in the presence of the stimulus. It is one of the most effective ways of building trust with an animal when the human is the aversive stimulus. In a busy veterinary practice, staff members are often not aware of how their body movements or proximity to the patient can cause distress. If the veterinarian and staff become aware of subtle signs of fear in the patient, then they can move more thoughtfully, gradually allowing the animal to get used to them.

Box 5 describes a strategy for reinforcing an animal for relaxed behavior instead of aggressive behavior. The whole process can take less than 5 minutes with many patients. It can be done during the history-taking part of the examination while the

---

Box 5
Strategy for reinforcing calm behavior

1. Start at a distance at which the animal shows relaxed or calm behavior.

2. Approach gradually. Observe the animal for a slight fear response (alertness, stillness, eyes widening, lean away, body tension)

3. Stop the approach when the slight fear response is noted. Wait calmly for a few seconds until some behavior indicative of relaxation is observed. (For example, eye lids relax, body tension decreases, shows interest in the surroundings, ear position relaxes.)

4. Take a small step back or lean away from the animal to reinforce the calm behavior by removing the aversive stimulus of human presence.

5. After a few seconds advance slowly until the slightest signs of fear are observed again and repeat Steps 2 and 3.

6. When close enough, place a preferred food item where the animal can reach it but not so close the placement of it causes an increased fear response.

7. Eventually offer the animal a preferred food item from your fingers or small container. Be careful not to push the food into the animal's personal space, but rather allow the animal to make a choice to reach out and take the food by choice.

When the animal is showing behaviors indicative of comfort for longer periods of time, it is then possible to begin training other behaviors.

---

animal's cage is on the examination table. At the very least, being aware of this approach will help the veterinary staff generally move with more care around small mammal patients.

Negative reinforcement is the learning principle at work when an animal behaves to remove or escape from an aversive stimulus present in the environment. In the strategy outlined (See **Box 5**) the animal is being taught that relaxation will cause the aversive stimulus to move away, rather than teaching only biting or running causes the aversive stimulus to be removed. In general, any time fear is escalating in an animal, it is best to stop approaching and give the animal time to assess and regain some sense of control over the environment. Then reinforce any behavior indicative of comfort by moving away from the animal and pausing briefly (negative reinforcement for calm behavior) before moving forward again.

Over time the animal will take a preferred food item directly as it learns to show relaxed behavior in close proximity to the person. Counterconditioning is a training strategy that attempts to change the reaction to an aversive stimulus from fear to pleasure. If desensitization and counterconditioning are used carefully, the animal will start to anticipate the presence of humans with pleasure and will eventually choose to approach people rather than immediately flee.

LOWERING PATIENT STRESS IN THE VETERINARY PRACTICE SETTING

There are many ways to reduce the anxiety level of small mammal patients in the veterinary practice setting. The following are some ideas for making the veterinary visit as stress free as possible.

1. Use and unscented cleanser to clean hands and examination table between patients. Lingering scents of other animals can create undesired responses. For example, ferret scent can elicit moderate to extreme fear responses in rabbits and rodents.

2. Cover the examination table with a towel or mat for noise reduction (banging instruments) and for patient comfort. Make folds in a towel for rodents to explore and use for hiding.
3. Avoid quick or erratic movements or speaking in a loud voice. Move slowly and talk softly.
4. Sit or stand relatively upright and avoid leaning over the patient.
5. Be prepared with instruments and supplies before restraining the patient.
6. Start with the least restraint possible and progress to more restraint only as needed.
7. Keep restraint times brief. It is better to restrain for a few seconds, release, and let the animal recover and then restrain again, rather than to restrain for long periods of time if the animal is struggling.
8. Allow the animal the illusion of escape when being restrained. Don't visually block all escape routes which may cause fear responses to escalate. Avoid covering the eyes at least initially.
9. Do not routinely put an animal on its back during examination. It is preferable to allow the back feet or hind end to have contact with something solid such as the table or a hand and lift the front legs only (**Fig. 1**).
10. If it is necessary to scruff an animal, allow the hind feet to rest on something solid.
11. Chemical restraint is preferable to using forceful physical restraint that results in extreme distress in a patient.

POSITIVE REINFORCEMENT TRAINING OVERVIEW

Once an animal is desensitized to human presence, further training can take place. The least intrusive and most positive method of training behaviors in small mammals

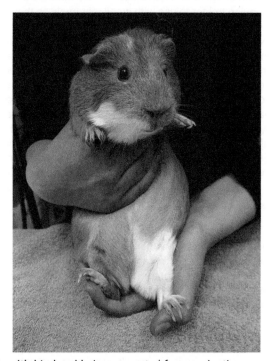

Fig. 1. Guinea pig with hind end being supported for examination.

is positive reinforcement training. Positive reinforcement training, in brief, is an operant conditioning process whereby something valuable to the learner is made available contingent on the performance of a desired behavior. For instance when a guinea pig is sitting calmly on the examination table, a small preferred food item can be offered to reinforce the calm behavior. Another example would be to offer a preferred food item when a small mammal patient looks toward a veterinary staff member. This will positively reinforce attention toward people and over time may result in the animal calmly approaching staff members, making it easier to handle the patient.

Shaping is the behavior modification procedure often used to train new behaviors. Shaping takes a behavior the learner is currently performing and gradually transforms it into the final target behavior by reinforcing small steps called approximations. An example would be training a rabbit to take medication out of a syringe. First the rabbit might be trained to look toward the syringe when presented, then to move toward and touch the syringe with its lips whenever it is presented. The next steps might include opening its lips on the syringe, then accepting a small amount of pleasantly flavored liquid from the syringe in its mouth and finally being able to take larger amounts of liquids from the syringe willingly.

A *bridging stimulus* or *event marker* is a training tool often used during shaping that can improve the communication between trainer and learner by making the contingency between the behavior and the reinforcer clear.

Good markers for small mammals are verbal, clickers and laser lights. Verbal event markers should be very short and clear such as "good" or "yes." The sound of a clicker can sometimes be frightening to a small mammal. The noise can be softened by holding the clicker in a pocket or using the top of a ball point pen initially. Laser lights are very helpful for deaf animals and they should be flashed close by in the animal's peripheral field of vision on the floor or on a wall. Tactile markers are not generally recommended for the novice trainer to use with small mammals as they can be perceived as threatening especially early in the training process.

When a trainer wants to evoke a behavior at will, then the behavior is given a *cue,* which is the stimulus or signal to the animal that they have an opportunity to perform the behavior for a reinforcing consequence. A cue can be a visual, acoustic, olfactory or tactile stimulus or combination of these.

If using auditory cues for small mammals they should be loud enough to be heard but not so loud as to startle. Many small mammals have poor long distance sight as well as a blind spot directly in front of them. If visual cues are used they need to be close to the animal's peripheral field of vision and involve small precise movements. Large rapid movements or objects that appear suddenly out of a blind area or from behind the animal can be perceived as threatening and should be avoided. For more detailed information on training, see the article by Heidenreich elsewhere in this issue.

WHERE TO TRAIN

Animals are learning about their environment every waking moment. Training can take place in a variety of settings. The home environment can be used to reinforce some simple behaviors such as a calm approach behaviors. These behaviors will increase in frequency by offering a preferred food item through the cage bars or open door several times daily, allowing the animal to approach and take the food. Speaking the animal's name just prior to offering the food is the beginning teaching a recall behavior using the animal's name as a cue.

When training a completely new behavior, it is helpful to set up a specific training area that has minimal visual, auditory, or olfactory distractions. The training area should be big enough that the animal can move away if it is afraid, but small enough that it is not difficult for the animal to maintain focus. Tabletops with a rubber mat for traction or a small wire pen on the floor are 2 examples of suitable training areas for small mammals. Training can also take place within the confines of the animal's enclosure. Once a behavior is fluent in the training location, then the animal should be moved to other locations where the behavior can be practiced under different circumstances and eventually becomes fluent under a variety of conditions.

A great place to train health care behaviors is at the veterinary clinic in the examination room. Veterinarians might consider scheduling time for clients to have access to an unused examination room for 10 or 15 minutes to conduct a short training session with their small mammal. For example clients can bring their animal's favorite food item and the client and staff can offer food for sitting on the exam table, getting on and off a scale, crawling through a towel, climbing into a hand, taking oral fluid, or being touched.

REINFORCERS

A stimulus is a reinforcer only if it maintains or increases the frequency of the behavior on which it is contingent. Reinforcers are always in the eye of the beholder and it is a good idea when training to have more than one reinforcer available as there are a number of variables that will change the value of a reinforcer on a daily basis. Common reinforcers for small mammals include food, touch, access to specific areas, objects, or other members of their social group.

Valued foods are the most common reinforcers used in small mammal training. The animal's regular diet can easily be used. In fact, feeding the diet during training sessions is more enriching then just placing it in a bowl free choice. Training with positive reinforcement mimics the mental problem solving needed to forage for food. Parts of the diet, such as specific seeds in a rodent seed mix, may be of higher value and on training days these should be withheld and used for training only. To increase the value of any food item, it is helpful to train right before regular feeding times when the animal is naturally anticipating a meal. Starvation is not necessary to train and should never be used as a means to increase motivation for food.

Food reinforcers for small mammals should be very small. This is so the animal does not satiate too quickly and to allow many repetitions of the behavior in a training session. There may be times when food reinforcers cannot be used at the veterinary practice because the patient needs sedation or a fasting blood sample. In these cases tactile reinforcers can be used if the animal has been conditioned to these. For instance, rabbits, rats and guinea pigs often exhibit calm, relaxed behavior when light pressure or a short light, stroking motion is applied to the space between the eyes up to the base of the ears. Otherwise wait until it is safe to offer a food reinforcer after the medical procedure.

Food reinforcers can be delivered by hand or by other means such as a spoon, tongue depressor, chop sticks, large tweezers, or a small squeeze bottle (if liquid). Food items should be easily accessible to the trainer because ideally they should be delivered within 2 seconds after the behavior or the event marker. If food delivery is too slow, the animal will have trouble understanding the contingency between the behavior and the reinforcer and training may be more difficult (**Box 6**).

SUGGESTIONS FOR SPECIFIC FOOD REINFORCERS

Veterinary staff should routinely ask clients to bring in their animal's favorite foods for a veterinary visit. It is also a good idea for the veterinarian to keep an easily accessible

---

Box 6
Food reinforcer tips

- Use a variety of healthy foods including items from the regular diet.
- Cut food into very small pieces appropriate to the size of the animal.
- Train before rather than after a meal.
- Deliver the reinforcer within 2 seconds after the behavior is presented.

---

variety of food reinforcers at the practice so the staff can participate in counterconditioning and training patients (**Box 7**).

TRAINING SESSION

Learning is taking place every moment that the animal is conscious and there are many opportunities to positively reinforce behaviors observed throughout a veterinary visit or in the animal's home environment. If a behavior occurs that is desired, reinforce it as quickly as possible.

Box 7
Species-specific food reinforcers

Rabbits/Guinea Pigs/Chinchillas

- High fiber pellets
- Fresh greens and vegetables up to the animal's daily limit
- Liquid foods such as canned unsweetened pumpkin or squash, unsweetened fruit juice, unsweetened vegetable juice
- Treat foods (limit to 2 teaspoons total of any combination of foods listed below per 5 pounds of body weight per day)
  - Grains (whole oats, barley, plain popcorn)
  - Dried fruit with no added sugar (dried mango and papaya are often favorites) or fresh fruit (bananas)
  - Nuts: shelled, unsalted, and cut into small pieces

Small Rodents (hamsters, mice, gerbils, rats)

- Pelleted rodent food broken into tiny pieces
- Unsalted raw seeds or nuts and grains (as listed for rabbit)
- Unsweetened fresh or dried fruit or vegetables
- Liquid foods same as rabbits
- Mealworms: fresh (mini size) or dried

Ferrets

- Dried ferret food (moisten to allow for easier chewing)
- Cooked meat (chicken, turkey, organ meat, etc.) or eggs
- Fatty acid supplement in small squeeze bottle, syringe or on spoon (maximum ½ teaspoon a day/ferret)
- All meat baby food on a spoon or tongue depressor or in a syringe (diluted with water or meat broth)

Training sessions designed to shape new behaviors should be short for small mammals. Five- to 10-minute sessions work well. For the novice, a good way to keep the session reasonable for the animal is to count out 10 reinforcers, and when those are gone, the session is over. As the animal and trainer gain experience, sessions may go longer.

Behaviors become strong with many repetitions. Short frequent sessions such as once or twice a day are much more effective than one long session once a week. Spending 5 to 10 minutes to train at feeding time works well for small mammals.

SHAPING PLANS FOR BEHAVIORS

There are many ways to approach training any behavior on the health care behavior list (See **Box 1**). Training is a fluid process, and if a suggested shaping plan is not working, the plan can be changed. It is often necessary to go back a few steps and then forward in shaping plans. Avoid the use of aversives no matter what the plan. The success of the session is dependent on the trainer who should strive to set up the environment in a way that will help the animal be successful at understanding the desired behavior.

The behaviors listed in this section are those that clients can train at home to prepare their small mammals for a veterinary intervention. Many of the behaviors listed can be trained without an event marker. For the shaping plans in this section M/R refers to marking (M) the behavior as it happens and then reinforcing (R) within 1 to 2 seconds afterwards. Once a particular behavior is on cue and fluent, then the event marker is no longer used.

Many of the behaviors described have cues "built in" to the training and an additional cue is not absolutely necessary. In the previous example of training a rabbit to take medication from a syringe, the sight of the syringe is the cue for the rabbit to move toward the syringe and accept medication. No additional cue is needed to signal this behavior. If a specific cue is desired, make sure it is one that is easily perceived by the animal. The cue is added when the behavior is repeating to the point that the trainer can easily predict when the next behavior will be offered. Add the cue as the behavior occurs to pair it with the behavior.

SAMPLE SHAPING PLANS FOR SPECIFIC BEHAVIORS
Recall

USE: Finding animal, getting it to come out of a carrier or hiding place.

- Start close to the animal and present hand with a high value food item in close proximity. If the animal advances toward the food item, mark (M) the movement and reinforce (R) when the animal arrives at the food.
- For each repetition gradually increase distance the animal must move to get to the food item. Eventually phase out having food item in the hand. Present the hand without food and M/R for approach.
- For a small rodent, the recall could include stepping onto an open hand. This is trained the same way using one hand as the recall location and one for delivering reinforcers.
- CUE: Add the cue, which could be the animal's name followed by the word "here" when it is possible to predict the approach. M/R when the animal arrives at the hand.
- Practice in other areas and on different surfaces until behavior is fluent.

Crating

USE: Being comfortable in a carrier for transport or as holding area.

It is recommended to use carriers that come apart easily with clips not screws. Clear plastic carrying cases with a removable top are good for smaller rodents. This behavior can be taught using a target or by luring with food.

- Work in a small space. This makes it more likely the animal will investigate the carrier.
- Take the door off the carrier or if it is a plastic box, take off the top and put it on its side. Place a sheet of newspaper or a thin layer of familiar bedding on floor of the container. Place a few preferred food items in the carrier.
- M/R if the animal goes into the carrier. Use the recall behavior or lure the animal out of carrier with a preferred food item.
- After a few repetitions stop putting food items in the carrier. If the animal goes into the carrier anticipating food, mark for going in and reinforce with preferred food items inside the carrier. Call the animal out again and repeat process. Gradually increase the time the animal remains in carrier before calling out.
- CUE: Add a verbal cue or hand signal (such as pointing finger) when the action of going into the carrier can be predicted.
- Add the door but leave it open and continue training. Eventually close the door for short periods of time.
- Once the animal is comfortable in the carrier, gently lift the carrier with the animal in it for gradually increasing periods of time. M/R after each lift. Place the carrier down and allow the animal to leave after each repetition.
- Repeat the training in different rooms. Raise criteria by adding short trips in the car. Gradually increase length of time spent in a carrier traveling in a car.

Targeting

USE: Targeting is used to teach a myriad of movement and stationary behaviors. Targeting is training an animal to touch a body part to a particular object. For example, nose to target stick, feet to side of cage (stand up), paw on hand for nail trim, going under, over, around, in and out of various objects (scale, carrier, exam table, etc.)

Targeting the nose to an object is usually the easiest first targeting behavior to teach small mammals. Target objects for small mammals might include commercial target sticks used for dogs or cats, thin dowels with a small ball at the end, chopsticks with a white or black tip (for contrast), fingers, spoon, pencils, etc.

- Start by putting the target on the ground and M/R if the animal investigates it.
- Gradually move the target up higher and M/R for orienting toward or touching the target with the nose NOTE: Close orientation to the target is often accepted criteria. It can be difficult or uncomfortable for some small mammals to make direct nose contact with the target.
- Move the target stick gradually to different positions. (up, down, left, right) M/R for each orientation.
- The presentation of the target stick becomes the cue for the behavior. An additional cue is not needed.

TARGETING ONTO A SCALE

Teach nose targeting and use the target stick to prompt the animal to move toward and then onto the scale. M/R for each successful approximation toward this goal.

- Increase the intervals of time on the scale between delivery of reinforcers. Use target stick to prompt the animal to move off the scale. Reinforce for getting off scale as well.

- CUE: The presence of the scale itself can eventually become the cue to present the behavior of getting on the scale.
- NOTE: This behavior can also be taught using a preferred food item as a lure to get the animal on and off the scale.

Stand on Hind Legs

USE: Being able to see the underside of the animal for an examination.

- Teach nose targeting and gradually move the target stick higher in small approximations to prompt the animal to stand on its hind legs. M/R each approximation.
- If the animal cannot stand on its hind legs, this can be trained near the side of a cage so the animal can hang onto the bars.
- CUE: The position of the target stick can be the cue.

Sit in a Box

USE: Gives the animal a familiar place to sit on the table during an examination (**Figs. 2** and **3**). Use a small low-sided box in which the animal can turn around. If using a clear box for rodents, it can also be examine the ventral side of the animal. This reduces the amount of time physical restraint may be needed (see **Figs. 2** and **3**).

- Place box in the training area with a few preferred food items inside. M/R for approaching the box. Eventually only M/R for getting in the box as described in the carrier training shaping plan.
- Give reinforcers while in the box to increase duration.
- M/R for staying in the box when it is picked up or moved.
- CUE: The sight of the box is the cue to get into the box. Therefore it is a good idea not to have the box present in the environment other than when the animal is expected to enter the box.

Oral Medication

USE: Preparing the animal for the eventuality of oral medication.

- Use an empty syringe as a target stick and M/R if animal touches it with its mouth.
- Put flavored water or feeding solution in syringe. When animal touches syringe push out a tiny amount of fluid, then remove syringe and M/R. Gradually increase

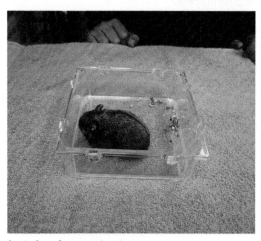

Fig. 2. Hamster in plastic box for examination.

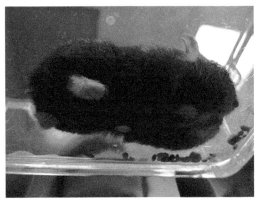

Fig. 3. Hamster seen from underside in clear plastic box.

the amount of fluid that can be given. Use fluid that is palatable see **Box 7** for ideas on liquid foods to use.
- CUE: The presentation of the syringe is the cue to present the behavior.

Towel Handling

USE: Being able to restrain animal in a towel for examination.

- Put a small towel in training area with large raised folds the animal can investigate (for large rabbits you can make a tunnel by draping a towel between two objects taller than the rabbit initially) Put preferred food items inside the folds or tunnel.
- M/R animal for investigating and then eventually going into a fold or tunnel.
- Apply gentle brief pressure to the animal's body while in the towel and M/R for calm behavior during touching. Gradually increase the length of time and pressure of the touch before M/R.
- Eventually try to gently lift the animal an inch off the table and replace on table and M/R. Gradually increase time and height animal is picked up.

CUE: The presence of the towel can be the cue for the opportunity to interact with the towel for preferred reinforcers.

Tactile Examination

USE: Being able to touch different areas of the animal's body for examination. The desired behavior is for the animal to stay relaxed during the examination.

- While the animal is in a relaxed state, lightly and briefly touch its back. This is an area that is usually not as sensitive as other areas. M/R for an interval of time in which touch is applied. The duration of the touch should be short enough that it does cause the animal to react.
- Gradually increase pressure and duration of touch and M/R each approximation.
- Over time work with other areas of the body in the same manner, starting with a light brief touch gradually increasing pressure and duration. M/R each time touch is applied and the animal remains calm.
- If the animal tries to flee when touched, do not M/R rather stop, remove the hand and wait until the animal exhibits calm behavior. Repeat the process but use light brief touch then M/R. Reinforce only for calm behavior and avoid pressuring the animal to respond with flight or aggression.

CUE: Add a verbal cue right before touching the animal. Over time some animals may find the touching pleasant and reinforcing in itself.

OTHER POSITIVE REINFORCEMENT OPPORTUNITIES IN THE VETERINARY PRACTICE

There are many opportunities to use positive reinforcement to continue the training that a client may have started at home or to train the animal to be comfortable with veterinary procedures. Veterinary staff should routinely ask clients to bring in their companion animal's favorite foods and the practice should have a variety of food items in portable containers easily available as well. Clients should be asked to refrain from putting food in the transport carrier or cage (other than what might be needed for getting the animal in the container for transport) to increase the motivation to take food from a staff member. The behaviors that the animal knows should be noted on the patient file so the staff can reinforce those behaviors during a visit or hospitalization.

Unless the animal needs to fast for a specific diagnostic test or for sedation, the positive experience can start at the reception desk by having the receptionist drop a piece of food into the carrier or cage as the client is checking in. See **Box 8** below for more ideas on how to use positive reinforcement in the veterinary practice environment. The veterinary staff should be cautioned to avoid offering reinforcement when the patient is exhibiting behaviors associated with discomfort. Instead staff can look for and reinforce calm and friendly approach behavior.

CLIENT EDUCATION

Information on training can be presented to the client in the form of handouts and videos. **Box 9** includes suggestions for a new client training packet. The veterinarian should consider building a library of short videos on training. Interested staff or an outside trainer that uses positive reinforcement methods can help develop these videos.

Box 8
Positive reinforcement opportunities during a veterinary visit

1. Reception desk: Receptionist drops a treat in carrier/cage during check-in.

2. Examination room: Open carrier on exam table. Scatter a few treats on table and allow the animal to explore prior to examination.

3. Reinforce any relaxed stationary behavior or nonaggressive approach behavior while animal is on the table. Use food or use tactile contact that the client has indicated the animal prefers.

4. Use food to lure the patient onto a scale for weighing. Give preferred food items while on the scale.

5. For small rodents, put a paper cup on its side in the cage with a preferred food item inside. When the animal is in the cup, lift the cup and animal out of the cage.

6. Offer preferred food items before and after the examination.

7. Have staff members drop preferred food items into a container at the front of hospitalized animal cages when passing by or visiting patients.

8. Find out what behaviors the animal has been taught and cue those behaviors a few times during an exam, or several times a day for a hospitalized animal. Performing familiar behaviors may lower the patient's stress in an unfamiliar setting. Put the list of known behaviors on an information card near the cage.

Box 9
New client training packet contents

- Reference list for training and behavior information including websites, videos and books
- List of local and national species-specific organizations
- Criteria for appropriate carriers and sources for purchase
- Information on what to routinely bring to a veterinary visit including preferred food items, food cup, stationing box, towel from home, and target stick
- Instruction sheet on desensitization and counterconditioning as methods of building a relationship with the animal and preparing for a physical examination
- Instruction sheets on how to train recall, targeting, stationing, and oral medicating

---

SUMMARY

A combination of health care behavior training in the patient's home and desensitization, counterconditioning, low-stress handling techniques, and positive reinforcement for desired behaviors in the veterinary practice will greatly reduce the level of anxiety and fear a small mammal will experience during veterinary intervention. These techniques will produce a patient that will choose to participate calmly in its own health care. In addition a bond of trust will be built between the patient and the veterinary staff and the bond between the caregiver and the animal will remain intact.

SUPPLEMENTARY DATA

Supplementary data related to this article can be found online at doi:10.1016/j.cvex. 2012.06.007.

REFERENCES

1. Yin S. Introduction. In: Low stress handling, restraint and behavior modification of dogs and cats: techniques for developing patients who love their visits. Davis (CA): CattleDog Publishing; 2009. p. 17–26.
2. Clay AW, Bloomsmith MA, Marr MG, et al. Habituation and desensitization as methods for reducing fearful behavior in singly housed rhesus macaques. Am J Primatol 2009;71(1):30–9.
3. Laule GE, Bloomsmith MA, Schapiro SJ. The use of positive reinforcement training techniques to enhance the care, management, and welfare of primates in the laboratory. J Appl Anim Welf Sci 2003;6(3):163–73.
4. Savastano G, Hanson A, McCann C. The development of an operant conditioning training program for new world primates at the Bronx Zoo. J Appl Anim Welf Sci 2003;6(3):247–61.
5. Crowell-Davis SL. Use of operant conditioning to facilitate examination of zoo animals. Compend Contin Educ Vet 2008;30(4):218–9, 223, 236.
6. Laule G, Whittaker M. Enhancing nonhuman primate care and welfare through the use of positive reinforcement training. J Appl Anim Welf Sci 2007;10(1):31–8.
7. Owen Y, Amory JR. A case study employing operant conditioning to reduce stress of capture for red-bellied tamarins (Saguinus labiatus). J Appl Anim Welf Sci 2011;14(2):124–37.
8. McKinley J, Buchanan-Smith HM, Bassett L, et al. Training common marmosets (Callithrix jacchus) to cooperate during routine laboratory procedures: ease of training and time investment. J Appl Anim Welf Sci 2003;6(3):209–20.

9. Bassett L, Buchanan-Smith HM, McKinley J. Effects of training on stress-related behavior of the common marmoset (Callithrix jacchus) in relation to coping with routine husbandry procedures. J Appl Anim Welf Sci 2003;6(3):221–33.
10. Heidenreich B. How to train medical behaviors. In: Proceedings of Association of Avian Veterinarians; 2006.
11. Friedman SA. Living and learning with animals course. October 2009. Available at: www.behaviorworks.org.
12. Fisher PG. Ferret behavior. In: Bradley Bays T, Lightfoot T, Mayer J, editors. Exotic pet behavior: birds, reptiles, and small mammals. St Louis (MO): Saunders Elsevier; 2006. p. 163–205.
13. Bradley Bays T. Guinea pig behavior. In: Bradley Bays T, Lightfoot T, Mayer J, editors. Exotic pet behavior: birds, reptiles, and small mammals. St Louis (MO): Saunders Elsevier; 2006. p. 207–38.
14. Evans E. Small rodent behavior: mice, rats, gerbils and hamsters. In: Bradley Bays T, Lightfoot T, Mayer J, editors. Exotic pet behavior: birds, reptiles, and small mammals. St Louis (MO): Saunders Elsevier; 2006. p. 239–61.

Training Birds and Small Mammals for Medical Behaviors

Sara Mattison, BS, MMin

KEYWORDS

- Operant conditioning • Birds • Small mammals • Medical behavior
- Positive reinforcement • Husbandry behavior

KEY POINTS

- Operant conditioning can be applied by animal caretakers to successfully train medical behaviors.
- Training birds and small mammals to perform behaviors that facilitate medical examinations can reduce stress for the animals, caretakers, and veterinarians and reduce the risk of injury.
- Training birds and small mammals to perform a variety of behaviors can result in improved preventative medicine regimens because they are easier to implement.
- Some medical behaviors take very little time to train, whereas others may take more time and effort.

INTRODUCTION

Operant conditioning with a focus on positive reinforcement is commonly used in zoos and aquariums to train zoo animals to perform a variety of behaviors on cue. These behaviors can be used to educate the public, facilitate daily husbandry tasks, enrich the animals' lives, and expedite medical care. At Point Defiance Zoo & Aquarium (PDZA), keepers in several different areas of the zoo have trained a myriad of medical behaviors. Articles published in conference proceedings and publications of the Animal Behavior Management Alliance, the International Association of Avian Trainers and Educators, and the American Association of Zoo Keepers, among other organizations, indicate they are not alone. The impetus to train animals to participate in their own medical care is to reduce stress for animals, their caretakers, and veterinarians. A reduction in stress leads to better recovery, more-accurate physiologic values, an increase in the overall health of captive animals,[1] and more-frequent applications of preventative medicine.

Because the science that zookeepers use to train parrots, raptors, rodents, and monkeys can be used just as effectively on animals that are kept as pets or for

Wild Wonders Outdoor Theater, Point Defiance Zoo & Aquarium, 5400 North Pearl Street, Tacoma, WA 98407, USA
E-mail address: Sara.Mattison@pdza.org

Vet Clin Exot Anim 15 (2012) 487–499
http://dx.doi.org/10.1016/j.cvex.2012.06.012
vetexotic.theclinics.com

research purposes, insight into the training of medical behaviors in a zoologic setting may provide inspiration or guidance for animal caretakers in many different fields.

Although the level of difficulty of training an animal to participate in its own medical care is related to the personal history and prior learning experience of both animal and trainer, some behaviors are generally easier to train than others. Medical behaviors can be divided into 3 categories: foundation behaviors, intermediate behaviors, and advanced behaviors.

- Foundation behaviors are those that are usually easy to train and are often useful in a variety of ways. They typically do not require a large time commitment to establish and can be maintained during routine husbandry. Examples include crate and scale training.
- Intermediate behaviors may require a longer amount of time to train. Once established, they are maintained by practicing the behavior regularly but less frequently than foundation behaviors. Examples include voluntarily participating in nail trimming and restraint procedures.
- Advanced behaviors may require a longer amount of time to train and may require a strong history of positive reinforcement to maintain the behavior. These behaviors often involve requiring the animal to endure a small amount of pain or discomfort. Examples include training an animal to accept an injection or masking for anesthesia without restraint.

FOUNDATION BEHAVIORS
Kennel Training

At the Wild Wonders Outdoor Theater (WWOT) at PDZA, nearly all of the animals are trained to enter and exit a kennel or crate. These animals are used in educational programs and need to be comfortable traveling in a kennel. Learning to calmly enter a kennel and stay there for a period of time has been relatively easy for most of the animals in the collection to learn. Kennel training can facilitate veterinary medicine in numerous ways. Crate training allows the following:

- Transport to the veterinarian
- Anesthesia in which the kennel acts as a chamber
- Anesthesia in which the kennel limits animal movement and allows for an injection
- Observation of the animal as it goes under and recovers from anesthesia
- Observation of the general physical condition of the animal

At WWOT, kennel training often begins the day an animal joins the collection. Kennel training is generally a combination of classical conditioning, in which the kennel is paired with preferred food items independent of the behavior of the animal, and operant conditioning, in which appropriate behavior by the animal is marked with a bridging stimulus and reinforced with preferred food items.

Shaping Plan for Training an Animal to Enter a Kennel

- Place the kennel in the enclosure. The kennel may be left outside of the enclosure if the animal exhibits any overt signs of discomfort with its presence. The door of the kennel is either closed, removed, or propped open so that it cannot accidentally trap the animal inside the kennel.
- Put part of the animal's normal diet near the kennel. Offer additional pieces of food when the animal approaches the kennel.
- Put the normal diet in the front of the kennel.

- Put the normal diet in the back of the kennel.
- Touch the door while the animal is inside kennel. Whistle and offer a preferred food item from outside of the kennel.
- Close the kennel door part way. Open the door. Whistle and offer a preferred food item from outside of the kennel.
- Close the kennel door all the way. Open the door. Whistle and offer a preferred food item from outside of the kennel.
- Close the kennel door all the way. Wait a few seconds. Whistle and offer a preferred food item from outside of the kennel.
- Close the kennel door all the way. Increase the amount of time the animal spends inside of the kennel before it is reinforced.
- Touch the outside of the kennel while the animal is inside. Whistle and offer a preferred food item from outside of the kennel.
- Move the kennel a short distance. Whistle and offer a preferred food item from outside of the kennel.
- Move the kennel a longer distance. Whistle and offer a preferred food item from outside of the kennel.

After enough repetitions, the behavior will become fluent. Smaller approximations and/or changing the arrangement can be used for animals that show a fear response to the kennel. For example, a trainer may take the door off the kennel or even take off the top of the kennel. Different styles of kennels may be used. Making the kennel more appealing by using different substrates or changing its color may also help.

One caveat about using a kennel to facilitate medical examinations is to make sure that most of the crating sessions result in desired consequences. For example, if the only time a bird is kenneled is to bring it to the veterinarian for an uncomfortable procedure, the bird may choose to avoid entering the kennel. At WWOT, entering a kennel is part of the animal's daily routine. Many animals enter and exit a kennel twice a day. Approximately 1 time in every 6 months of crating may result in being anesthetized. The adverse effect of this one experience will be outweighed by the approximately 350 times it ended in something neutral or desired.

Scale Training

Scale training is another behavior that is generally easy to train an animal to do. Training strategies may vary because animals and scales come in many different shapes and sizes. A scale fitted with a t-perch can be used for birds (**Fig. 1**), whereas a flat perch can accommodate an animal trained to stand directly on it (**Fig. 2**) or while in a crate (**Fig. 3**). Some scales are specially designed to accommodate larger birds (**Fig. 4**).

Scale training is particularly important for birds. Bird body condition is difficult to visually evaluate. Many species of birds are adept at hiding signs of illness, and a drop in weight is often the first observable indication of a potential health problem.

Scale training is a variation on stationing or targeting. A tawny frogmouth (*Podargus strigoides*) was trained to stand on a scale after more than 15 years of being caught and placed in a cardboard box to be weighed. Instead of grabbing the bird (which was very comfortable around humans), the trainer put a hand up to the bird's feet and touched them gently. The bird responded by lifting a foot and placing it on the hand. By slowly lifting her hand upward, the trainer encouraged the bird to step entirely onto her hand. Desired food items were offered to the bird when it stood calmly on the hand. The bird quickly learned to step onto the hand to receive the preferred food items. The trainer was then able to place the bird on a t-perch on a scale and get an accurate weight with no stress to the bird or the trainer.

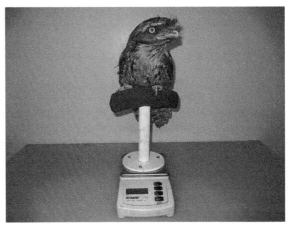

Fig. 1. A tawny frogmouth (*Podargus strigoides*) stands on a scale fitted with a t-perch. (*Courtesy of* Maureen O'Keefe.)

For larger birds and mammals, a scale with a flat surface is often used. An Abyssinian ground hornbill (*Bucorvus abyssinicus*) was trained to step onto any perch that the trainer pointed to in its enclosure (**Fig. 5**). The perches in the enclosure were changed regularly. The bird learned to step onto short stumps, tall stumps, large polyvinyl chloride tubes with flat tops, and many different branches. Because the bird was trained to station on many different types of objects, stepping onto a flat scale was not a difficult transition, even though it had a shiny metal surface and provided less traction than the normal stations.

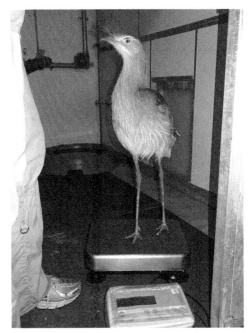

Fig. 2. A red-legged seriema (*Cariama cristata*) stands on a flat scale. (*Courtesy of* Maureen O'Keefe.)

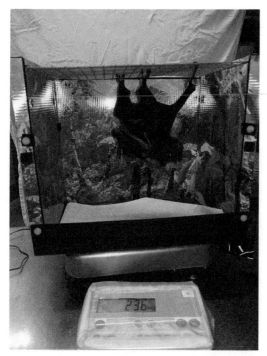

Fig. 3. A giant Indian fruit bat (*Pteropus giganteus*) is weighed on a flat scale while resting comfortably in its crate. (*Courtesy of* Maureen O'Keefe.)

INTERMEDIATE BEHAVIORS

Training an animal to stand on a scale or enter a kennel can be valuable. These two behaviors enhance husbandry and medical care and are generally easy to train. However, there are some behaviors that are more involved but still worth the investment of time.

Voluntary Nail Trims

Many types of animals are frequently brought to the veterinarian to have nails trimmed. Often the animal has to be restrained. The nails may have over grown, which may make it difficult to avoid cutting into the quick. The animal may show fear responses or aggressive behavior in response to the procedure. The potential stress associated with this can be avoided by training the animal to allow its nails to be trimmed without restraint.

A North American porcupine (*Erethizon dorsatum*) was trained to allow its nails to be trimmed (**Fig. 6**). The porcupine was already trained to target, walk from point A to point B across a stage, go into a kennel, and participate in walks on zoo grounds. The animal had a long history of positive-reinforcement training with its trainers. This history facilitated training the animal to allow nail trimming without restraint.

Shaping plan for training a porcupine to allow nail trimming

- Introduce the nail trim station. The nail trim station includes a high bar and a low bar. The high bar is for the placement of the front feet. The low bar is for the placement of the back feet.

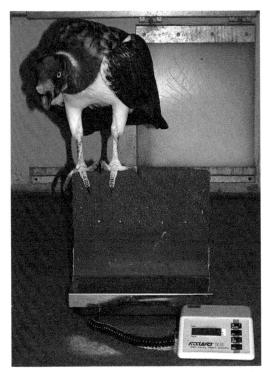

Fig. 4. A king vulture (*Sarcoramphus papa*) stands on a large bird scale. (*Courtesy of* Karen Povey.)

- Bridge and offer a preferred food item for approaching the nail trim station.
- Bridge and offer a preferred food item for putting the front feet on the top bar. Because the porcupine frequently stood on its hind legs to receive food items, the posture was easily captured.
- Bridge and offer a preferred food item for lowering the hindquarters while the front feet remain on the top bar.
- Bridge and offer a preferred food item for moving the hind feet toward the bottom bar while the front feet remain on the top bar.

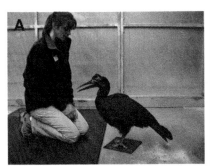
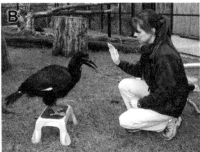

Fig. 5. (*A, B*) An Abyssinian ground hornbill stands on a variety of stations including a flat mat and a step stool. (*Courtesy of* Karen Povey.)

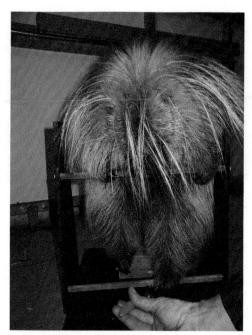

Fig. 6. A North American porcupine (*Erethizon dorsatum*) stands on a station to allow its nails to be trimmed. (*Courtesy of* Maureen O'Keefe.)

- Bridge and offer a preferred food item for all 4 feet on the appropriate bars.
- Touch the nail with nail clippers. Bridge and offer a preferred food item for maintaining the position. Trim the tip of the nail. Bridge and offer a preferred food item for maintaining the position.
- Trim multiple nails. Bridge and offer a preferred food item for maintaining the position.

Several training challenges were presented. The first was that the porcupine showed more sensitivity about its right front paw being manipulated than the rest of its feet. The animal tended to hold food in that foot. Extra time was required to desensitize that foot to touching. The second occurred when the trainer cut into the quick of one of the nails. Fortunately, this did not occur during the initial stages of training. The nail bled and had to be cauterized to stop the bleeding. The behavior was reestablished after a few weeks of retraining. The long positive-reinforcement history with nail trimming helped the trainers quickly recover the behavior.

Allowing Manual Restraint

Many species of birds are restrained for medical behaviors. A towel or sheet is placed over a bird's head and body. The head and body are firmly held. For raptors that are trained and handled for educational programs, toweling is often done while the bird is standing on the glove. Other birds may be captured in midflight or while they are standing on a perch or the ground. This maneuver often requires dexterity and good spatial skills on the part of the handler. Training a bird to maintain position and allow a towel to be wrapped around its body results in an efficient, effective, and less stressful restraint process. At PDZA, a green-wing macaw (*Ara chloroptera*) was trained to allow toweling while standing on a perch (**Fig. 7**).

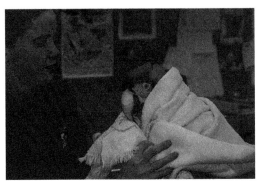

Fig. 7. A green-wing macaw (*Ara chloroptera*) allows a towel to be put around its body while standing on a perch. (*Courtesy of* Maureen O'Keefe.)

Shaping plan for training a parrot to allow restraint in a towel

- Present the towel in front of the bird that is stationed on a perch. Bridge and offer a preferred food item for touching the towel with its beak. (At PDZA, the bird had been previously trained to target with its beak. It was a simple transition from touching a target with the beak to touching the towel.)
- Hold the towel between the bird and the trainer so that the towel is just above the level of the bird's eyes. Offer the bird a preferred food item. Position the presentation of the food item so the top of the towel brushes the bird's head as it reaches for the treat.
- Lower the towel so that the towel blocks the line of sight between the trainer and the bird. Bridge and offer a preferred food item when the bird pushes its beak underneath the towel toward the trainer or target. Lower the towel so that the bird must duck its head underneath to orient toward the trainer or target. Allow the towel to slide down the bird's neck. Bridge and offer a preferred food item.
- Allow the towel to rest lightly on the bird's back for several seconds. Bridge, remove the towel, and offer a preferred food item.
- While the towel rests on the bird's back, slowly fold the sides in front of its chest. Bridge, remove the towel, and offer a preferred food item for maintaining the position.
- With the towel completely around the bird, the trainer gently presses on one wing. Bridge, remove the towel, and offer a preferred food item for maintaining the position.
- With the towel completely around the bird, the trainer gently presses on both wings. Bridge, remove the towel, and offer a preferred food item for maintaining the position.
- With the towel wrapped completely around the bird, the trainer gently presses on the back of the head. Bridge, remove the towel, and offer a preferred food item for maintaining the position.
- Wrap the bird in the towel, position hands around the wings and the back of the head, and lift up gently. Stop before the bird shows any signs of discomfort. Bridge, lower the bird back onto the perch, remove towel, and offer a preferred food item for maintaining the position.
- Wrap the bird in the towel, position hands around the wings and the back of the head, and lift up gently until the bird lets go of the perch with its feet (**Fig. 8**). Stop before the bird shows any signs of discomfort. Bridge, lower the bird back onto the perch, remove the towel, and offer a preferred food item for calm behavior.

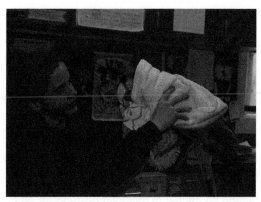

Fig. 8. A green-wing macaw is lifted off of its perch while wrapped in a towel. (*Courtesy of Maureen O'Keefe.*)

ADVANCED BEHAVIORS

Advanced behaviors may take more time to establish and may be difficult to maintain because they often involve an element of discomfort. Because of this, trainers may want to evaluate if training these types of behaviors is an effective use of time. If an animal has to undergo medical procedures on a regular basis, it might be reasonable to train it to cooperate in the procedure. If the animal is healthy and only needs infrequent medical attention, it may not be practical to spend time training advanced behaviors. Each situation should be evaluated based on the veterinary needs of the animal and the amount of time and number of staff available to train. If an animal has a solid history of learning behaviors through positive reinforcement, advanced behaviors may be easily trained and may be useful for medical care.

Stand for Injection

Many animals have been conditioned to stand calmly and maintain a position for an injection at WWOT. For some, this is an extension of a station behavior. For others, it is something that the animal allows because of its long-term relationship with the caretaker. A Canada lynx (*Lynx canadensis*) at WWOT requires subcutaneous injections twice monthly. The animal has been handled on a daily basis in its role as a program animal since it was several weeks old. The lynx allows its handlers to administer the injection either while lying in the bottom half of a kennel filled with straw in its enclosure or while out on walks around the zoo grounds. The animal does not respond to food as a reinforcer but it is receptive to companionship and attention from staff members. This attention is paired with injections and has allowed staff members to provide the animal's treatment without restraint. Similarly, a clouded leopard (*Neofelis nebulosa*) allows staff to give the animal an intramuscular injection to anesthetize the leopard for its annual physical examination. Staff members can enter the enclosure to administer the injection. One staff member uses gentle touching to reinforce calm behavior. During touching, the trainer can gently scruff the animal's neck to momentarily restrict movement. The other staff member then gives the injection in the animal's flank. The cat is permitted to walk away through a shift door into another enclosure, which allows staff members to safely exit the enclosure.

Some staff members do not have a relationship that allows them to enter the enclosure. They have been successful giving the cat an injection through the mesh of the enclosure. When the cat approaches the mesh, one staff member scratches the animal on the head. This practice usually results in the cat pressing its body against the fence, allowing the second staff member to give the injection in the flank.

Training an animal to stand for an injection can also be done with animals that do not have comfortable relationships with their trainers. Using a barrier and shaping the behavior with small approximations can result in a successful injection procedure for small cats. Depending on the animal's comfort level, a barrier may not be required. Trainers will want to evaluate the animal and the environment to determine the safest option to successfully train the behavior.

Shaping plan for training an animal to maintain position for an injection

- Train the animal to go to a station.
- Give the cue to go to the station and then touch the animal on the part of the body that will receive the injection. Bridge and offer a preferred food item for maintaining the position and for calm behavior.
- Give the cue to go to the station and then touch the animal with a capped syringe. Bridge and offer a preferred food item for maintaining the position and for calm behavior.
- Give the cue to go to the station and then touch the animal with a syringe with the blunted needle tip. Bridge and offer a preferred food item for maintaining the position and for calm behavior.
- Give the cue to go to the station and then touch the animal with the regular needle tip. Bridge and offer many preferred food items for maintaining the position and for calm behavior.
- Give the cue to go to the station and then give the injection. Bridge and offer many preferred food items for maintaining the position and for calm behavior. If this is an injection for anesthesia, noningestible reinforcers may be required, such as tactile or enrichment items.
- Most training sessions should not involve actually inserting the needle, even after that step has been reached. Regular sessions whereby the animal only feels the blunt needle tip will help maintain the behavior.

Many animals respond well to adding another signal just before touching with the needle. A word like pinch or touch can indicate that the injection is about to happen. The animal can then choose to move away and not participate or stand still to receive the available reinforcers.

Voluntary Anesthesia

Some animals can be trained to allow a mask to be placed over the face for anesthesia. The green-wing macaw (*Ara chloroptera*) at WWOT that was trained to be toweled was also trained to place its head into a mask for anesthesia (**Fig. 9**).

Shaping plan to train a parrot to participate in masking for anesthesia

- Show the mask to the parrot. When the parrot touches it with its beak, bridge and offer a preferred food item.
- Hold the mask with the open side toward the parrot. Bridge and offer a preferred food item when the parrot touches the inside of the mask with its beak.

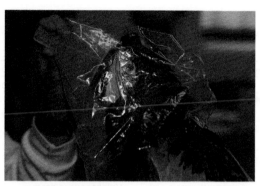

Fig. 9. A green-wing macaw puts its beak into a funnel while being trained for voluntary anesthesia. (*Courtesy of* Maureen O'Keefe.)

- Place a plastic bag over the mask. Fold it back to allow a small part of it to protrude beyond the mask. Bridge and offer a preferred food item when the parrot touches the inside of the mask with its beak.
- Unroll the plastic bag to allow it to protrude farther beyond the mask. Bridge and offer a preferred food item when the parrot touches the inside of the mask with its beak.
- When the parrot has its head inside the mask with the plastic bag around its neck, touch the back of the neck or head gently. Bridge, remove the mask, and offer a preferred food item.
- When the parrot has its head inside the mask with the plastic bag around its neck, tighten the plastic bag around the neck and/or back so that the bag will not leak. Hold the wings against the body. Bridge, remove the mask, and offer a preferred food item.
- When the parrot has its head inside the mask with the plastic bag around its neck, introduce a second person to work around the parrot to simulate turning on the anesthesia. Bridge, remove the mask, and offer a preferred food item.
- When the parrot has its head inside the mask with the plastic bag around its neck, turn on a small amount of oxygen. Bridge, remove the mask, and offer a preferred food item.
- When the parrot has its head inside the mask with the plastic bag around its neck, introduce the anesthetic gas. Hold the wings against the bird's body and support the back of the head while the anesthesia takes effect.

At PDZA, the green-wing macaw trained for the procedure would sit comfortably wrapped in a towel and place its head into the anesthesia mask. The towel was added to this procedure because training with the anesthetic agent was infrequent. In the event that the bird showed discomfort with the procedure, the towel allowed the trainer to securely hold the parrot as the gas started to take effect.

MEDICAL BEHAVIORS IN LITERATURE

A review of conference proceedings and articles from animal care professional organizations shows that a wide variety of behaviors can be trained in an even wider variety of animals **Table 1**.

Table 1
References of behaviors that can be trained

Common Name	Scientific Name	Behavior	Citation
Red-crowned cranes	*Grus japonensis*	Defecate on cue	Donahue[2]
Gentoo penguin	*Pygoscelis papua*	Scale training	DeLorenzo[3]
White-naped crane	*Grus vipio*	Artificial insemination	Crowe[4]
Red-cockaded wood pecker	*Picoides borealis*	Weigh	Conk[5]
Magellanic penguin	*Spheniscus magellanicus*	Semen collection	O'Brien et al[6]
Tawny eagle	*Aquila rapax*	Voluntary eye drop procedure	Mangum[7]
Birds	Various	Oral medications	Vine[8]
Green-wing macaw	*Ara chloroptera*	Voluntary anesthesia	O'Keefe et al[9]
Red-legged seriema	*Cariama cristata*	Stand for radiographs	Mattison[10]
Mangabey	*Cercocebus chrysogaster*	Diabetes management	Dawn et al[11]
North American river otter	*Lontra canadensis*	Enter induction tube	England[12]
Flying fox	*Pteropus spp*	Weights, nail trims, medications	Alm & Dougall[13]
Tamandua	*Tamandua tetradactyla*	Stationing	Hernandez & Morgan[14]
Spotted hyena	*Crocuta crocuta*	Blood draw	Morrell & Murray[15]
Francois' langur	*Trachypithecus francoisi*	Encouraging maternal care	Shephard[16]
Douc langur	*Pygathrix nemaeus*	Weights, hand injection	Halko-Angemi[17]

SUMMARY

A wide variety of captive animals can benefit from being trained to participate in their own medical care. Operant conditioning is a powerful tool for animal care takers because it allows a complex medical behavior to be broken down into simple steps that can then be reinforced. Operant conditioning works for any desired behavior, whether it is jumping through a hoop, vocalizing on cue, or standing for an injection. From standing on a scale to allowing a blood draw without restraint, medical behaviors are within reach. With a long enough reinforcement history, cooperating in medical care can be as stress free to present as any other trained behaviors in an animal's repertoire.

ACKNOWLEDGMENTS

Special thanks to Karen Povey (Associate Curator of Conservation and Education, PDZA), Maureen O'Keefe (Senior Keeper, WWOT), Jessica Sutherland (Staff Biologist, WWOT), and Adrienne Umpstead (Staff Biologist, WWOT) for training many of the behaviors discussed here as well as contributing their insights to this article and helping the author with revisions.

REFERENCES

1. Stoskopf MK. The physiological effects of psychological stress. Z Biol 1983;2(3): 179–90.
2. Donahue K. Red-crowned crane behavior modification training, vol. 11. Laughlin (NV): ABMA Wellspring; 2010. p. 25–9.
3. DeLorenzo K. Gentoo training: introducing twelve penguins to operant conditioning. Chicago: American Association of Zoo Keepers; 2006.
4. Crowe CR. Artificially inseminating white-naped cranes. Philadelphia: American Association of Zoo Keepers; 2010.
5. Conk CV. Vertical is the way to go! How to obtain a weight on a red-cockaded woodpecker. Galveston (TX): American Association of Zookeepers; 2007.
6. O'Brien JK, Oehler DA, Malowski SP, et al. Semen collection, characterization, and cryopreservation in a magellanic penguin (*Spheniscus magellanicus*). Z Biol 1999;199–214 Wiley-Liss.
7. Scot M. Tawny eagle (*Aquila rapax*) voluntary eye drop procedure, vol. 18. Clermont (FL): International Association of Avian Trainers and Educators; 2011.
8. Catherine V. From shows and zoos to show in zoos. Clermont (FL): International Association of Avian Trainers and Educators; 2005.
9. Mattison SM, O'Keefe M, Povey K. From inspiration to action: reaching new heights with new ideas. Clermont (FL): International Association of Avian Trainers and Educators; 2006.
10. Mattison SM, O'Keefe M, Povey K, et al. From stage to stethoscope: the evolution of a behavior. Laughlin (NV): Animal Behavior Management Alliance; 2007.
11. Dawn S, Jason W, Dennis P. Management of a diabetic golden-bellied mangabey (*Cercocebus chrysogaster*). Philadelphia: American Association of Zoo Keepers; 2010.
12. England M, Animal Behavior Management Alliance. Obstacles in training: a look at overcoming adversity to achieve success, vol. 12. Laughlin (NV): ABMA Wellspring; 2011. p. 18–22.
13. Alm V, Dougall A. Using operant conditioning training to aid in health care practices for flying fox. Salt Lake City (UT): American Association of Zookeepers; 2008.
14. Hernandez ML, Laura M. Daily husbandry and training of a diabetic tamandua (*Tamandua tetradactyla*). Salt Lake City (UT): American Association of Zookeepers; 2008.
15. Laura M, Murray M. Training two separate behaviors to draw blood from 2.0 spotted hyena. Philadelphia: American Association of Zoo Keepers; 2010.
16. Shepard T. Innovative methods to encourage mother infant bonding in the rare Francois' langur, trachypithecus francoisi francoisi. Philadelphia: American Association of Zoo Keepers; 2010.
17. Halko-Angemi A. How training and understanding behavior were used to medicate and evaluate a terminally ill douc langur, vol. 9. Laughlin (NV): ABMA Wellspring; 2008. p. 9–11.

Working Raptors and Veterinary Medicine
Preserving the Client/Veterinarian Relationship

Rebecca K. O'Connor

KEYWORDS

- Falconry • Positive reinforcement • Applied behavior analysis • Anthropomorphism
- Raptors • Body language

KEY POINTS

- Understanding the basics of falconry and the needs of clients with working raptors, whether in educational, rehabilitation, or falconry situations, can be critical to the client/veterinary relationship.
- Clients managing working raptors have a more complicated relationship with their birds of prey than most other animal owners.
- Falconry has a long history that has engendered entrenched ideas of the handling and care of raptors, and an understanding of training with positive reinforcement can be helpful to the client/veterinarian relationship.
- Repercussions from aversive experiences in working raptors can be extensive and create problem behaviors in raptors that are difficult to resolve.

INTRODUCTION

The art and practice of falconry has been in existence for more than 3000 years, originating in the Middle East and spreading throughout the East. It eventually made its way to Europe, where it was dubbed, "the sport of kings," and has a rich history of traditions, tools, and superstitions. It is a technique of bringing meat to the table that arose in a time before firearms were invented; thus, it is no surprise that the literature and beliefs of falconry are deep-seated even today.

Falconry has a history in nearly every continent and culture. Each species, with its slightly different physiology, temperament, and quarry, has its own set of techniques, equipment, and history in falconry. Manuals on the training of raptors, such as the Holy Roman Emperor Frederick II's *De arte venandi cum avibus* (*The Art of Hunting with Birds*), written between 1244 and 1248, are still read and considered useful to falconers today. Thus, it is fair to say that many techniques and beliefs in falconry,

Animal Behavior Consultant, 31 Ensign Street, Banning, CA 95817, USA
E-mail address: rebecca@blueskywriting.com

Vet Clin Exot Anim 15 (2012) 501–511
http://dx.doi.org/10.1016/j.cvex.2012.07.001
1094-9194/12/$ – see front matter © 2012 Elsevier Inc. All rights reserved.

which are also used in the rehabilitation and educational use of raptors, are entrenched and even at times antiquated (**Fig. 1**).

Modern falconry, although not as pervasive as in times when a trained raptor was a reasonable proposition for a meal, exists in a larger population than might be imagined. In the middle of the twentieth century, falconry experienced a renaissance throughout Western Europe and in North America, and today there are a few thousand licensed falconers in the United States.[1(p131)] Owning and hunting a raptor, however, for the purposes of falconry requires extensive licensing in the United States that necessitates an apprenticeship, passing a test, and inspection of facilities where the raptor is housed. These rigorous regulations equate to a knowledge base and an opinion base that may have more depth and doggedness than owners of nonregulated animals have. Throughout this article, the term, *working raptors*, is used to be inclusive of all raptors that are being handled and trained, even if they are not in falconry situations. A raptor that is to be released back into the wild without training may not need the level of consideration discussed in this article. Keeping a relationship with a client who trains raptors to be in a working relationship requires understanding the relationship, prejudices, and requirements of a falconer.

UNDERSTANDING RAPTOR BEHAVIOR

Raptor behavior can be subtle and different from that of the prey species of birds that people commonly keep as pets. Having a basic understanding of behavior and body language can keep examinations and treatments from undermining a falconer's relationship with a raptor. It is important to understand the basic requirements of keeping a raptor calm and at ease (**Fig. 2**).

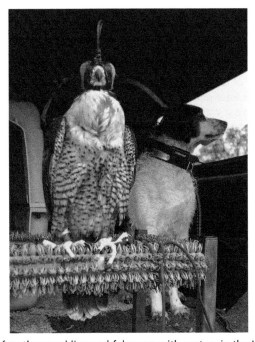

Fig. 1. There are a few thousand licensed falconers with raptors in the United States today.

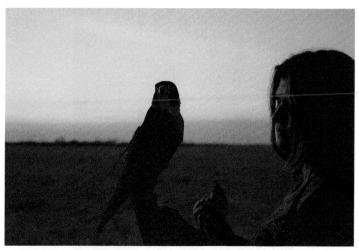

Fig. 2. Falconers' birds are often comfortable being hooded.

Hooding

Falconry hoods are handmade for individual birds of prey. Head shape and size, which vary not only between species but also greatly between genders, require the perfect match for each bird. A well-fitting hood completely covers a bird's eyes without letting in any light while not rubbing on the cere or against the eyes.[2(p81)] Because raptors are visually stimulated, raptors that are hooded are relieved of stimulus and manage stressful situations with greater ease. Not all falconers hood their birds, but a bird of prey that hoods is more likely to remain calm. With this understanding, it is best to keep a raptor's hood on for as much of the examination as possible, and falconers appreciate this.

Handling

Mishandling of a raptor has greater implications than with most animals in veterinary care. Most animals that interact with veterinarians are not expected to fly great distances and return of their own volition, a request that requires a long history of positive reinforcement and as few aversive experiences as possible. A raptor that has experienced enough aversive experience with humans may no longer wish to fly back to its falconer and, therefore, no longer be a workable falconry or show companion. In a rehabilitation bird, it may also negate the possibility of training to hunt proficiently before release, which requires falconry techniques. With this understanding, being sensitive to how a raptor handler likes a veterinarian and staff to interact with the bird can be helpful to a raptor's overall health or recovery.

As Webster note in *North American Falconry and Hunting Hawks*, a seminal edition to falconry literature, a raptor should rarely be touched without permission to do so: "Many birds are quite intolerant of handling even by their owner, and will either fight or panic at any such liberty from a stranger."[2(p291)] Although the idea of getting "permission" from a raptor is anthropomorphic, understanding that each raptor has been trained in a specific way and that mishandling may create setbacks in training can go a long way toward helping relationships with both handler and bird, both of which may make a difference in treatment and recovery (**Fig. 3**).

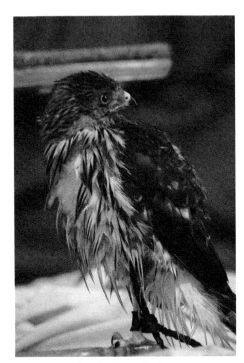

Fig. 3. Imprinted juvenile Cooper's hawk after a bath.

Passage Versus Imprinted

Working raptors either come into human care as chicks or as young adults and their expected behavior can be drastically different depending on their experience. A raptor that has been raised by humans before fully feathered is considered *imprinted*. A raptor that has come into human care after being fully feathered but before its first molt is considered a *passage*. With the exception of rehabilitation situations, a working raptor is almost never taken into human care as an adult. In falconry, a bird like this is considered a *haggard* and generally undesirable for training. The amount of time a raptor has spent in the wild can greatly determine the comfort level a raptor has with its handler and especially with strangers.

Depending on the species and age of its first human handling, raptors can manage examinations with more or less duress. For example, a falcon that has been raised by humans beginning at a few weeks of age may experience little stress when being handled physically by a stranger. An imprinted bird is generally at ease with humans and with handling. A falcon of the same species and even the same gender that has been taken or forced by circumstances from the wild as an adult finds any experience with unknown humans more stressful.

Behavior, comfort level, and training techniques can be vastly different depending on species, in passage birds as well as in imprinted birds. Certain species, such as those in the genus *Accipiter*, are more prone to stress, and even an imprinted bird can be prone to undesirable behavior after an aversive experience with humans. A young bird, not yet fully feathered and at an age when it is absorbing and learning from every interaction, can also be reactionary to coercive interactions. Training a raptor can be time consuming and tedious, requiring strict adherence to creating positively reinforcing experiences. The tremendous setbacks that might be experienced by a traumatic experience in a veterinarian's office can be frustrating to a client. Every raptor that comes into a veterinarian's office should be considered a new handling experience and the advisement of the client in handling requirements can make the visit a less stressful event for all parties involved.

Body Language and Applied Behavior Analysis

Understanding raptor behavior and positive reinforcement training basics can have a great impact on successful medicine and clinic visits. Although many raptor handlers make basic assumptions about their birds with broad brush strokes, as with any animal, the key to understanding behavior is applied behavior analysis (ABA) and body language. Having an understanding of behavior analysis as applied to raptors and what a raptor's body language looks like can help a manage examinations, suggest means of treatment, and assist a raptor trainer who is struggling.

Individuals who have learned to read raptor body language are more sensitive about maintaining a relationship based on trust with their birds, and veterinarians who approach behavior with raptors this way create less stress on the animals and perhaps can even assist handlers in bettering their relationships with the raptors. Many of the training techniques falconers have used historically involve flooding, such as the traditional means of manning. Although flooding can create fast results and works, it is not training birds to do anything other than acquiesce. By watching body language, a raptor handler can allow a bird to express discomfort and can handle the raptor appropriately. A bird that learns the human interacting with it will back off when it raises its hackles or opens its mouth is more likely to give a warning before it engages in aggressive or other undesirable behavior. Traditional manning, which involves simply exposing a bird to situation until it "gets over it," can teach a bird that body language is ignored and useless as a means of communication. Overall, positive reinforcement is the most important tool in a raptor trainer's arsenal.

To effectively use ABA, a baseline ability to read behavior is required. Veterinarians with a basic understanding of raptor behavior can gauge the comfort or stress levels of birds in their care and react appropriately. Knowledge of body language enhances this further. Paying attention to eye shape, feather positioning, and displays of basic behavior reveals the level of stress a raptor is exhibiting. It can also help in diagnosis if there is an understanding of whether a raptor is engaging in normal activity (**Tables 1** and **2**).

Table 1	
A brief overview of raptor body language indicative of comfort	
Body Language	**Description**
Stretching	Extending one wing and simultaneously stretching foot
Preening	Running feathers through beak; look especially for bird engaging preening gland at base of tail
Bathing	Standing in bath pan, dunking body in water
Turning head upside down	Turning head 180° to look at something
Investigating	Examining surroundings with active interest
Puffed beard	Feathers below the beak puffed out
Relaxed eyes	Eyes oval but not almond-shaped
Rousing	Raising all feathers and shaking them back into alignment
Feaking	Rubbing beak on perch, glove, or other as if to clean it
Foot up	Standing on one foot with other raised and tucked in feathers

Table 2
A brief overview of raptor body language indicative of stress and/or illness

Body Language	Description
Slicked feathers	Feathers are tight against the raptor's body
Looking for escape route	Bird looks around for a place to escape
Bating	Bird jumps off perch to length of leash in an effort to escape; excessive bating toward the falconer can also be a sign of stress in the form of excessive hunger
Rowing wings	Raptor sits on the perch and flaps wings
Wide eyes	Eyes are perfectly round
Gaping mouth	Mouth is wide open for an extended time
Gular flutter (owls)	Feathers at throat flutter in and out
Sudden change in normal behavior	Bird does not present expected normal behavior, such as reacting to the presentation of food
Wing tips below tail	In resting state, wings fall below tail, a sign of conserving metabolic energy
Blank stare	Bird looks into distance and does not focus on environmental stimuli
Extraordinary tameness	Bird does not respond to unusual environments or environmental changes in which it would normally show signs of stress, instead appearing calm
Flicking food	Instead of eating, raptor touches food with beak and flicks food away
Fluffed feathers, no response	Bird has no interest in interacting
Overall appearance	Change in care of plumage (also look for a fading in color of new growth of talons)
Lowered head	Head down below shoulders
Rapid respiratory rate	Breathing rate is more rapid than normal

ANTHROPOMORPHISM AND ANIMAL VALUE IN WORKING RAPTORS

Grasping the complicated relationship and emotions tied to managing a working raptor can be helpful to a veterinarian working with an injured hunting partner. Although falconers are attached to their working partners, it is often a long investment of time and attachment that also includes an understanding that nature is red in tooth in claw and that most raptors are killed on the job. Also, most falconers are pragmatic about the attachment their raptors might have toward them. T.H. White, a writer more famous for his novel, *The Once and Future King*, than for his memoir, *The Goshawk*, summarized it well: "The thing about being associated with a hawk is that one cannot be slipshod about it. No hawk can be a pet. There is no sentimentality."[3(p212)] In short, falconers tend to not be anthropomorphic toward their birds.

A pragmatic approach, however, does not assuage devotion and a feeling of tremendous investment in a falconer's charge. Trust, although not as tactile as the adoration of dogs or cats, is still hard won with birds of prey. There is a level of pride and a deep attachment that occurs through the long process of developing trust with a raptor. Add to this the degree of licensing and requirements that must be met in order to own a bird of prey in the United States and falconers may have strong opinions and expectations about the care of their birds. In this way, not much has changed from the times of the Emperor Frederick II of Hohenstaufen, who wrote, "Without an experienced teacher and frequent experience of the art properly directed no one, noble or ignoble, can hope to gain in a short time an expert, or even ordinary knowledge of falconry."[4(p6)] Falconers have in-depth knowledge about the handling, habits, and needs of their raptors. Although they may seem more detached about the care, involving them in evaluation and treatment can be helpful to both raptor and the client relationships.

RAPTORS IN THE EXAMINATION ROOM

Raptor handlers are often an excellent source for diagnosis, minimizing stress to the raptor and for assisting the veterinarian. This is especially true of falconers. Falconers handle their birds on a daily basis, weighing them, checking the state of the muscle on their keel, checking their feet, and examining their urates and feces and, overall, examining the condition of the hawk or falcon before taking it into the field to fly. To a falconer, all these things are hints to the physical shape and potential attitude of a raptor. A bird in excellent condition is more likely to hunt well and return to the caregiver when cued.

Falconers' knowledge of the baseline behavior and appearance of raptors in their care can assist greatly in gathering information to diagnose what is ailing a raptor. Many falconers keep meticulous records and chances are falconers have logs of daily weights and behavior to consult or share with a veterinarian. Falconers are often adept at recognizing signs of coccidiosis, aspergillosis, yeast infections, sour crop, and many other common ailments. Some diseases are more common in certain species, and falconers are also likely to be familiar with the challenges of the particular species with which they are working. They are also likely to recognize when something is wrong with their raptor that is subtle and bring the raptor in for diagnosis early. Falconers may not realize how helpful sharing the wealth of information they have can be in the examination room. It is an excellent idea to quiz a raptor's caregiver for information that can help in the preliminary considerations for diagnosis (**Fig. 4**).

Once a veterinarian begins an examination, it is an excellent idea to involve the falconer as well. There are many portions of the examination that a trained raptor tolerates without being grabbed and restrained, keeping the examination stress-free for the bird. Most falconry birds have been trained to step on a scale and allow palpation

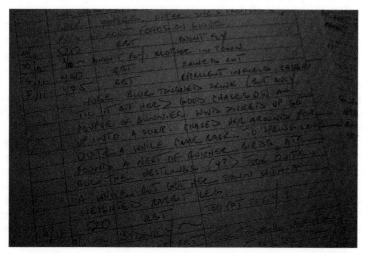

Fig. 4. Falconers often keep excellent records of their birds' weights and behaviors.

of the feet, keel bone, tail, and head. A bird that hoods can have the majority of the examination done while sitting on the glove, including a mouth swab with a calm raptor. If a raptor needs to be grabbed and restrained for blood draws or more invasive examination, it can be helpful to let the falconer do the restraining. A falconer is going to recognize immediately if a bird is overstressed and also is more familiar with the bird's behavior while under restraint. Most raptors are restrained now and then to change out their equipment and for grooming, so a falconer is likely to have a great deal of experience with a particular bird.

Out-of-office follow-up treatment of a raptor can also be kept low in stress to the bird if the veterinarian discusses training techniques that can help with aftercare management. Many falconry birds are only in the care of a falconer for 1 or 2 years and only handled for 5 months of the year, so training for medical treatment may not be something falconers are interested in pursuing. Many raptors are in educational situations or permanent captivity, however, and training for veterinary care is to the benefit of the raptors. Barbara Heidenreich noted that SeaWorld San Diego has used training to "treat a chronic bumble foot problem on an African fish eagle (Haliaeetus vocifer). Training the bird to accept the application of topical medication and bandage changes allowed the staff to avoid the difficult and stressful task of capturing and restraining the eagle on a daily basis. This bird was also conditioned to accept an intramuscular injection without restraint."[5] In the same way that falconers trains a hawk or falcon to accept wearing a hood, touching of the keel, and changing out equipment, they can train a raptor to allow injections, bandage changes, cloacal swabs, and oral medication.

HELPING CAREGIVERS HELP THEIR RAPTORS

As Michael McDermott states in his book, The Imprint Accipiter, "The most basic description of falconry ethics is 'to do right by the bird'."[6] It is fair to say that the majority of individuals who work with raptors wish to do what is best for the birds that are in their care and go to great lengths to provide excellent care. In the falconry apprentice system, however, novices are likely to find themselves learning from an unwilling or unpracticed teacher and struggling. The same may be true of individuals wishing to work rehabilitating raptors. Many individuals who have learned to work successfully with raptors have done so the hard way—through much trial and error as opposed to mentorship. Falconers do not tend to spend a great deal of time teaching and, as unpracticed teachers, often have difficulty describing training techniques and raptor body language. Rehabilitators may be in a similar situation if they work with few staff members or volunteers. With this in mind, veterinarians are in an excellent position to assist clients in consulting the appropriate resources and in learning some of the basics (**Fig. 5**).

Julie Ponder, DVM, notes in regards to her work with captive raptors, "the behavioral problems we see are the result of inadequate training or lack of understanding of birds' natural biology,"[6(p67)] confirming that it is generally agreed that competence in training techniques and an understanding of natural behavior are critical pieces of overall raptor health. Ponder also notes, "the rigors of the selection process for ownership of a captive raptor assures a client has baseline knowledge before acquiring a raptor.[6(p71)]" Although a legal possessor of raptors does demonstrate a baseline knowledge, it sometimes is to a novice's detriment because there is an assumption that tested knowledge of husbandry and care is enough. It is true that in order to receive a falconry license, an individual must demonstrate a basic understanding of raptor identification, common diseases, acceptable husbandry, and legislation. Body language and behavior are critical pieces of a raptor's well-being but are not required learning for

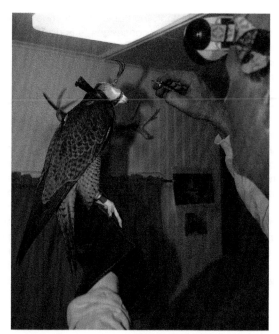

Fig. 5. Falconers' birds are often trained to sit on the glove for beak trimming and changing out equipment.

licensing, likely because falconry is a hands-on ongoing learning experience. Handling competence is not a factor in the procurement of falconry or other permits giving individuals permission to be in possession of raptors. It would be to the benefit of raptors for mentors, including veterinarians who have avian-focused practices, to make it a goal to assist novices in learning basic ideas that can be used in every training situation.

A trainer who is astute at reading raptor body language is well equipped to learn to apply the basics of ABA with an emphasis on positive reinforcement. A bird can be trained to interact with a falconer and to accept tactile interaction through positive reinforcement. More complex behaviors, such as flying high and waiting on, can also be trained.[7,8] Other behaviors that need to be shaped or eliminated can be addressed with ABA. Every behavior has an antecedent and a consequence. Through identifying what precedes and follows a behavior in question, a trainer can modify it. Understanding that a behavior that is reinforced repeats itself, a trainer is armed with the means to modify, encourage, or extinguish behavior. The applications for better husbandry and problem solving through ABA are immense and can start with some simple issues.

Behaviors as common as bating can be addressed by ABA. Bating is the act of jumping off a perch or glove in an act of escape that is stopped by reaching the end of the jesses and leash. Bating is a natural behavior, but intense ongoing bating is not natural, it is trained. Bating birds of prey can wear down or break feathers, damage their tarsi, or even break legs. Intense bating is an undesirable behavior. Many birds of prey, however, bate incessantly around feeding time.

The antecedent and consequence of a falcon's bating behavior can be ascertained by observing the behavior. In a falcon bating for food, the trainer's appearance, with hands behind the back, might be the antecedent and the consequence is the trainer stepping closer. To change the behavior, the trainer can change the antecedent or the consequence. In this case, changing the consequence is discussed.

The ultimate consequence is receiving the food, but just approaching may be a reinforcing consequence because the food gets closer. To cease reinforcing the bating, the trainer needs to stop approaching when the raptor is bating, choose another behavior to reinforce, and then methodically teach the falcon that this new behavior is a more effective means of getting food closer. A trainer might then reinforce the desired behavior by moving forward with the food only when the falcon is sitting upright on the perch.

When the trainer appears with the food and the falcon bates, the trainer should stop moving toward the bird and wait for the falcon to cease bating, jump back on the perch, and sit upright. After consistently ignoring the falcon's bating and only reinforcing the perched upright posture by moving forward, the falcon learns to stay on its perch waiting for the presentation of food. This is a simple example of a trained behavior that can make a tremendous difference to a raptor's mental and physical well-being if a handler understands ABA. It can also have applications when a raptor has injured a leg and bating can be problematic to recovery. Beyond understanding the requirements of creating the best possible experience in a veterinary visit, understanding the basic applications of ABA can be helpful to aftercare as well.

SUMMARY

With only a few thousand falconers in the United States, chances are most veterinarians do not have many falconers visiting their clinics. All the same, the basics of falconry are the groundwork for all training with educational, entertainment, and rehabilitation raptors. A basic understanding of the history, philosophies, and training involved in falconry can be helpful in working with birds of prey. More so, understanding the challenges and needs of clients who bring in working raptors can make the overall experience of the visit more pleasant for everyone.

A veterinarian who is well versed in the most recent advances in avian medicine but does not frequently work with working birds can strengthen relationships with falconers and similar raptor caregivers by understanding the challenges of training birds of prey and the obstacles that can create setbacks. Falconers may not always be studied in the most recent avian medicine and may even have antiquated ideas, but they have tremendous knowledge of raptor behavior, especially in the day-to-day behavior of their individual birds. A falconer may be an asset in diagnosing a problem.

Perhaps most importantly, falconry has a long way to go to slip away from the superstitions of training and embrace the science of applied behavioral analysis. In a world where apprentice falconers do not have to get their information from ancient books or the rare falconer they might stumble on and a world where the Internet offers myriad opinions, veterinarians can facilitate making falconry not just an art but also a science. The more veterinarians are versed in ABA and the benefits of positive reinforcement, the more allies raptors and new falconers will have to this advanced and valuable way of thinking. The future of falconry is exciting and veterinarians can play a large part in shaping it.

REFERENCES

1. Peeters H, Peeters P. Raptors of California. Berkeley (CA): University of California Press; 2005.

2. Beebe FL, Webster HM, Enderson JH. North american falconry & hunting hawks. 4th. Denver (CO): North American Falconry & Hunting Hawks; 1964.
3. White TH. The Goshawk. New York: Viking Press Inc; 1951.
4. HohenStaufen, F II. The art of falconry. [trans.] Casey A. Wood and F. Marjorie Fyfe. Stanford: Stanford University Press, 1943.
5. Heidenreich B. Training birds for husbandry and medical behavior to reduce or eliminate stress. Association of Avian Veterinarians Conference. 2004.
6. McDermott M. The imprint accipiter. Self Published; 2008.
7. Hess L. Avian behavior: an evolving discipline (round table discussion). J Avian Med Surg 2007;22(1):66–72.
8. Pryor K. Click: falconry and modern operant conditioning. California Hawking Club; 2001.

Teaching Avian Patients and Caregivers in the Examination Room

Ellen K. Cook, DVM

KEYWORDS

- Positive reinforcement • Parrot • Behavior • Veterinary • Physical examination
- Targeting • Toweling • Medicating

KEY POINTS

- Animal behavior is infrequently addressed by the veterinarian in clinical practice.
- Companion parrot behavior is that of wild, not domesticated, species.
- Parrots presented in a veterinary setting often avoid touch or examination.
- Using positive reinforcement techniques can enable the veterinarian to handle parrots more effectively.
- Veterinarians can teach these techniques to parrots and caregivers during a routine examination setting.

 A video of target training accompanies this article http://www.vetexotic. theclinics.com/

INTRODUCTION

"First, do no harm." Veterinary professionals are all familiar with this essential axiom in the art of veterinary medical practice. Veterinarians are trained as scientists. They are taught to observe objectively, weigh and measure all normal and abnormal conditions in their patients, perform appropriate testing, diagnose disease, perform surgery, and prescribe treatment. This all works well in theory but the reality of providing care for companion animals, especially birds, presents many obstacles.

Working with species of parrots that are intelligent, undomesticated companions make veterinarians' efforts quite challenging. Many avian patients, with good reason, show extreme fear responses toward people associated with veterinary care. Many clients report that their relationship with their birds has suffered serious damage as a result of attempting to medicate and treat a variety of conditions. The patient

Cicero Veterinary Clinic, 210 South Peru Street, Cicero, IN 46034, USA
E-mail address: ellendvm@aol.com

Vet Clin Exot Anim 15 (2012) 513–522
http://dx.doi.org/10.1016/j.cvex.2012.06.011
1094-9194/12/$ – see front matter © 2012 Elsevier Inc. All rights reserved.

survives the disease process — but at what cost to the human-bird bond? At what cost to the veterinarian-client-patient relationship?

Veterinarians face the problem of communication with their patients and also with their clients. Veterinarians seldom adequately address the challenges of client compliance and actual patient aftercare in the home. Goals of veterinary professionals should match those of the companion animal caregivers: providing the best and simplest husbandry practices and treating diseases effectively and safely.

Clients are exposed to various resources in this age of information technology that help and hinder a veterinarian's effort to provide care for a patient. The outdated information and mythology on avian behavior still available today can have strong repercussions for veterinary care. These often result in patients who have learned fear responses or aggressive behavior in response to humans' attempts to interact. The resources listed and references cited in this article are ones the author recommends as the most reliable, humane, and easiest teaching methods available.

LEARNING ABOUT TRAINING

To prepare for teaching clients, veterinary professionals must familiarize themselves with the basic principles of behavior analysis with an emphasis on positive reinforcement. The most comprehensive and reliable resources now available for learning about avian behavior include the following:

- Echols, M. Scott, DVM. Captive foraging: The next best thing to being free. Zoologic Education Network, 2006. http://avianstudios.com/products/captive-foraging-dvd/
- Friedman, Susan G., PhD Living & learning with parrots: the fundamental principles and procedures of teaching and learning. Online course. www.behaviorworks.org
- Heidenreich, Barbara. Books, DVDs, Good Bird Magazine and more. www.goodbirdinc.com
- Johnson, Melinda. Getting started: clicker training for birds. Sunshine Books, Inc, 2004. http://store.clickertraining.com/clforbi.html
- Morrow, Linda. Clicking with birds: clicker training your companion parrot: a beginners guide. 2002. http://www.avitrain.com/manual.html
- Pryor, Karen. Don't shoot the dog: the new art of teaching and training. Bantam Books, 1999. http://www.clickertraining.com/?source=sthplog

Just 13 years ago there were very few resources on avian behavior. The only resources available focused on information gathered from anecdotal experience. None of these avian behavior resources were very effective or humane in resolving the most common undesirable behaviors in companion birds. All resources in this article detail the science of behavior analysis and the mechanics of positive reinforcement training in a format easily understood and accessible to anyone interested in parrot behavior.

The principles of behavior work with all species of animals (including humans). Some effort and perseverance is necessary to understand the concepts and how to apply them. However, the value of understanding the science of applied behavioral analysis cannot be underestimated. At the very least, veterinarians can become familiar with the practical application of positive reinforcement training. They then can then easily introduce this concept to clients during a visit to the clinic with their companion parrot (See the articles by Heidenreich and Farhoody elsewhere in this issue.).

TARGET TRAINING DURING AN APPOINTMENT

Targeting is recommended as the initial behavior to teach using positive reinforcement (**Fig. 1**). Targeting is used as the basis for many other behaviors and for teaching husbandry behaviors, including grooming, medicating, handling, and so forth (For more information on targeting see *An Introduction to the Application of Science Based Training Technology*). Chopstick, straws, spoons, balls, or foot toys are frequently used by the author as targets for birds (**Fig. 2**).

In the examination room, cotton-tipped applicator sticks may include targets; most birds show an interest in exploring the bit of cotton at the end of the stick with their beaks. The bird is then reinforced, usually with very small pieces of a preferred food item, each time it touches the target. Clients are asked to bring their birds' most preferred food items, which have been withheld from the bird for a day or two before their appointment. Veterinarians can also keep a variety of food items commonly preferred by avian patients in the examination room (**Fig. 3**). **Table 1** lists preferred food items for different species based on the author's experience.

See Heidenreich's article, *Pick a treat, any treat*, for additional information on various types of preferred reinforcers for different parrot species.[1]

Although a client may find it odd to train a parrot to touch a stick, veterinarians can explain that target training is basic communication between teacher and student. It does not take long for a parrot to learn that touching the stick results in desired consequences. This is of special significance for wild animals kept in captivity. The caregiver controls the environment. Targeting gives the bird a choice, a chance to act on its environment: touches the target, desired things happen; does not touch the target, nothing (good or bad) happens. If the bird wants the particular items offered as reinforcers, it will continue to touch the target object. Giving animals the choice to participate is hugely empowering for the captive wild animals. Veterinarians can emphasize this point to the caregiver.

Discussing and teaching targeting to a patient and client can happen before the bird is examined. This can help to relax the client and give the patient time to desensitize to the environment. It also allows the veterinarian to begin developing a trusting relationship with the patient based on desired outcomes instead of aversive experiences. Target training also allows the veterinarian to perform a thorough visual examination of the patient and observe bird-caregiver interactions. Veterinarians can schedule wellness appointments for 30 minutes to allow time for discussion of husbandry and

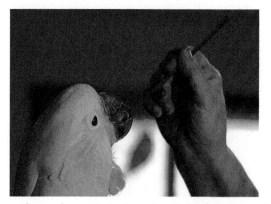

Fig. 1. A Moluccan cockatoo demonstrates targeting its beak to the end of a stick.

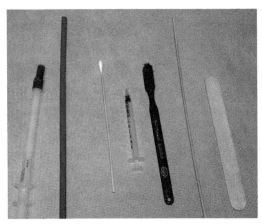

Fig. 2. Objects commonly used as targets for avian patients.

behavior topics, the physical examination, and diagnostic testing. During a young cockatiel's first veterinary visit, the author demonstrated target training. The bird learned to target in less than 3 minutes (See Video 1 online [within this article at www.vetexotic.theclinics.com, September 2012 issue]).

Many parrots exhibit some degree of hand avoidance because of previous learning experiences, especially in the veterinary office. These birds benefit greatly from target training in the examination room. Veterinarians can interact positively with the bird before approaching with hands. Clients often comment that their bird is "better behaved" or "not as scared" (interpreted as: the bird exhibits less screaming, flailing of wings, and biting) as during previous veterinary visits when training with positive reinforcement is part of the process.

PROCEDURAL APPROACH

Avian patients can learn that each interaction with the veterinarian results in desired outcomes or, at the very least, does not involve aversive situations. This is especially

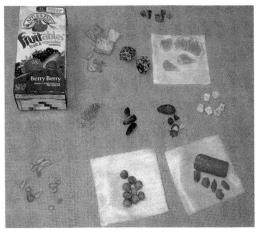

Fig. 3. Commonly preferred food items of avian patients.

Table 1
Most commonly preferred food items for use in training

	Budgerigar Cockatiel Parrotlet	Conure Mini-Macaw Pionus	Amazon	African Gray	Cockatoo	Macaw
Seeds Millet, hemp, sunflower, flax, safflower	Millet	Millet	Sunflower	Sunflower	Sunflower	Sunflower
Nuts[a] Pine nuts, almonds, pecans, walnuts	Pine Nuts	All Nuts	All nuts	Almonds	Almonds	Pine Nuts Almonds
Fruit: Dried or fresh fruit in season	Apple Berries	Grape Berries	Apple Grape	Grape	Orange	Apple Grape
Vegetables: Dried or/frozen	Corn	Peppers	Corn Peas	Corn	Corn Peas	Corn
Other[b] Hand feeding formula, fruit juices	NA	Juice	Juice	Juice	Formula Juice	Formula Juice

[a] Nuts should be chopped into very small pieces.
[b] Birds that have been handfed when young will often take liquids readily from a syringe.

critical for avian veterinarians to remember. Many of the procedures commonly used to examine, diagnose, and treat various health issues in avian patients are perceived as aversive and coercive by the birds and their caregivers. Make no mistake—clients do not enjoy seeing veterinarians "manhandle" their beloved bird. When veterinary professionals exhibit concern about the patients' comfort and distress and attempt to alleviate discomfort, they will find caregivers more receptive and open to effective communication.

Acknowledging this fact gives veterinarians the opportunity to explore alternate methods of handling and focusing on treating patients in a more positive manner. By spending a few minutes before and after the examination or procedure offering preferred food items to the bird, veterinarians can offset some aversive associations occurring with some handling.

Most birds learn targeting very quickly. As soon as they understand the concept that touching the stick earns desired consequences, veterinarians can then introduce new target objects, such as the beak speculum, the light, and stethoscope, or whatever instrumentation will be used. This familiarizes the bird with these novel objects in a framework of positive reinforcement. This also provides an opportunity to teach the client that the use of targeting has practical applications beyond teaching the bird to simply touch a stick.

Veterinarians can use this process to introduce a tuberculin syringe as a target to the bird and explain how to teach the bird to readily take medicine from a syringe. Numerous clients report they had an excellent relationship with their companion parrot until the bird became ill. After repeated "swoop and grab" maneuvers, awkwardly wrapping the bird in a towel (awkward for the inexperienced), and forcing a syringe into the bird's beak, it is not surprising the bird learns to avoid its caregivers. Many other clients report they were only able to give one or two doses of medication to their birds. Providing the best veterinary care for avian patients includes teaching clients how to medicate their birds in a safe, easy, and positively reinforcing way for both caregiver and bird. Furthermore, clients appreciate the veterinarian's efforts to help them maintain their relationship with their companion parrot (**Fig. 4**).

It is important for the veterinary practitioner to be always cognizant of the basic wild nature of avian patients. Equally important, birds' visual acuity and sensitivity to being preyed on can make them highly vigilant in a veterinary setting. They can be quite attuned to the movements and activities of people around them. This necessitates special care in the veterinarian's movements and vocal tones and inflections around avian patients. Moving slowly and thoughtfully, speaking in low monotones is helpful when initially approaching the bird.

An examination can begin by opening the carrier door and allowing the bird to exit on its own or step up onto the caregiver's hand. The caregiver can be asked to place the bird on a stand or the top of the carrier. A bird on a perch will often more readily step up to the veterinarian or assistant than a bird that is on the caregiver's hand, arm, or shoulder. Sometimes favorite food items can be used to lure the bird to step onto the hand.

Many avian patients have had a history of aversive experiences with towels. Veterinary practitioners can question the caregiver about the birds' reaction to towels before bringing a towel into the bird's visual field. In the author's experience, minimal restraint works best with most avian patients. If a towel is necessary, the towel is shown to the bird and then placed on the lap or presented in a way to stimulate exploration, interaction, or play behaviors with the bird. In just a few minutes, many birds will at least tolerate being wrapped in the towel (**Fig. 5**).

It may be helpful for the veterinarian to sit and remain seated when examining the bird. The veterinarian should avoid staring directly at the patient. If possible, the practitioner can focus and orient toward the client and glance at the bird occasionally. When approached slowly, many birds will allow an examination without significant restraint.

Some preparation is necessary to minimize stress to the avian patient during the examination process. Necessary instruments and equipment to be used (eg, stethoscope, light, applicator sticks, microscope slides) should be made readily available.

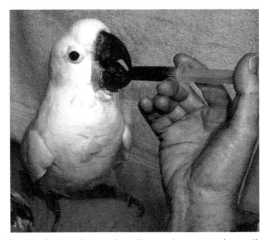

Fig. 4. Target training can be used to train avian patients to voluntarily accept medication from a syringe without restraint.

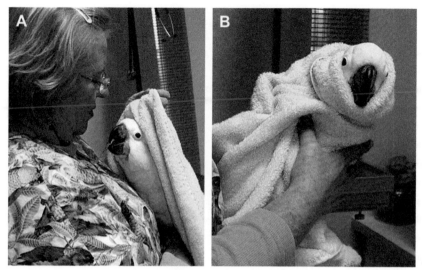

Fig. 5. (*A*) If a towel is necessary, the towel is shown to the bird and then placed on the lap or presented in a way to stimulate exploration, interaction, or play behaviors with the bird. (*B*) Many birds will at least tolerate being wrapped in the towel.

The veterinarian should outline the process for the client and plan for appropriate diagnostic testing (eg, venipuncture, cytology specimens) before touching the patient. The veterinarian and assistant can then handle the bird in a quick and efficient manner.

FOLLOW-UP

In the author's practice, clients are called 2 weeks after their appointment to inquire about the physical and behavioral condition of the bird. Clients are encouraged to work with targeting with their birds and to pursue further education about positive reinforcement training using the provided reading and online resources. During future appointments, teaching or refreshing the application of positive reinforcement are repeated (**Box 1**).

As a result of the increased interest in parrot behavior, there are some parrot behavior classes available in different areas. However, veterinarians should investigate these thoroughly before recommending them to clients. There are still many training and behavior consultants that routinely advocate the use of coercive techniques in all fields of animal training. Although positive punishment does work, undesirable fallout occurs.[2] This manifests itself primarily as increased aggressive behavior, apathy, and avoidance behaviors in companion parrots.

TRAINING CHALLENGING PATIENTS

Some avian patients exhibit extreme avoidance behavior toward hands and/or towels. Some patients are not motivated to accept preferred food items when at the veterinary hospital. There are other ways to interact successfully with these types of patients. Many of these birds still investigate the target stick and can be reinforced in other ways. Veterinarians can move away from the bird and increase distance from the patient or return the bird to the caregiver if those consequences are desired by the patient. Learning to read and interpret birds' body language and becoming familiar

Box 1
Behaviors clients can teach at home

Basic Behaviors

Targeting

Step up and step down onto a variety of perches

Step onto a scale or perch on a scale

Entering and leaving cage and/or carrier

Stepping onto new people

Toweling

Intermediate Behaviors

Taking liquids from syringe

Filing and/or trimming nails

Recall (walking)

Advanced behaviors[a]

Harnessing

Recall (flight)

Fun behaviors

Retrieve

Wave

Handshake

[a] Advanced behaviors should be taught by or with the assistance of an instructor experienced in using positive reinforcement techniques with avian species.

with species variations (ie, macaws' facial blushing) is vital to the avian practitioner (See Heidenreich's DVD, *Understanding parrot body language*).[3] Demonstrating sensitivity to a bird's body language makes it easier for veterinary professionals to predict and avoid aggressive behavior and fear responses. Practitioners can focus on doing things that facilitate the presentation of body language indicating comfort.

Scheduling additional time may be required for challenging patients. In some cases it is beneficial to have the client and patient visit the clinic and an examination room several times before the actual examination. These visits can be paired with preferred food items, attention, or other consequences the animal prefers. The amount of knowledge gained by a complete visual examination of the patient and a thorough history taken from the client is often underestimated. It may take three to four visits, with clients working with their birds at home, to be able to perform a physical examination on the patient. Once trained, targeting is also helpful in calming difficult patients. A bird that is familiar with the behavior can focus on doing the action and has prior history of it resulting in desired consequences. This can help associate pleasant experiences with visiting the veterinary clinic. Any patient presented in non–life-threatening circumstances can be better served with these techniques.

If the patient is in an emergent state, minimal stress is a requirement. Most of these birds are quiet and do not resist handling. Necessary treatment to stabilize the patient is provided as quickly as possible.

ADDITIONAL BENEFITS OF POSITIVE REINFORCEMENT TRAINING

In nearly 40 years of veterinary practice, the author has seen companion animals of all species abandoned, relinquished to humane societies, or euthanized because of the animals' undesirable behaviors. Companion birds, primarily parrots, are no exception to society's penchant for quick-fixes and avoidance of anything inconvenient, uncomfortable, or requiring effort. Life is disposable, cost does not matter: palm cockatoos and hyacinth macaws are found next to budgerigars and cockatiels in many parrot welfare facilities. Veterinarians lose a patient and client whenever a parrot loses its home because of undesirable behavior issues. It is in a veterinarian's best interest financially, ethically, and professionally to be aware of this situation, to proactively address clients' concerns about behavior, and to be able to provide some sort of assistance when undesired behaviors arise.

Common behavior problems presented by companion parrots include vocalizing excessively, aggressive behavior, and pterotillomania (feather damaging behavior). Some of these patients have an underlying physical disorder. Regardless of the presence or absence of medical disease, behavior serves a function for the bird, even those considered problematic. Clients often seek their veterinarian's assistance in resolving these issues. Consulting with veterinary behaviorists and/or professionals that specialize in avian behavior can be of help in such situations.

If veterinarians are unable to devote the time necessary to become familiar with basic behavior science, then perhaps a technician or assistant in the practice would have the interest and ability to learn and work with behavior with clients and their birds. In the author's practice, both the registered veterinary technician and veterinary assistant are trained in the basics of positive reinforcement training techniques. This has expedited appointments by giving the veterinarian time to focus on addressing the medical condition that precipitated the appointment. If this is not feasible, it is recommended clients are directed to the list of aforementioned resources.

It is important for veterinarians to understand that positive reinforcement works with all species, including humans.[4] Teaching clients positive reinforcement training techniques gives veterinarians the opportunity to observe client behavior and to positively reinforce their actions. Humans often find verbal praise to be high-value reinforcement. In the examination room it is important to look for opportunities to reinforce a client's behavior. For example, praising a client for training their parrot to stand on a scale may result in good weight records for the life of the bird. Teaching people is much like training parrots. It is important to set them up for success, ignore undesired behaviors, and always reinforce desired behaviors. This works as well with clients as it does with animals. Veterinarians will find it builds trust with the client, just as it does with the patient.

SUMMARY

Many veterinarians do not find behavioral issues to be personally or financially rewarding. However the behavioral health of avian patients cannot be ignored. Avian caregivers are very concerned with all aspects of their birds' health and veterinarians need to address their increasing awareness of these issues. There are increasing numbers of examples demonstrating the use of positive reinforcement training techniques during examinations of patients in the small animal veterinary field. However, there are few resources available for the companion avian veterinarian. Fortunately, positive reinforcement and the associated science of applied behavioral analysis are applied across species lines. This means resources that focus on learning theory in general are suitable for avian species. Although not every individual or situation lends itself to training during a veterinary examination, in many cases stress can be reduced by focusing on a simple behavior such as targeting. For over 10 years, the author has regularly incorporated positive reinforcement training techniques during avian wellness appointments. This has led to clients expressing an interest in learning more and to the development of classes and resources as additional services offered to clients with companion parrots. Reinforcing clients and birds can lead to trusting relationships for all involved. The result of spending a few minutes listening to clients, responding to patient behavior, showing them that their relationship is of value, and demonstrating a desire to help, is a satisfied client with a strong bond to the veterinarian and practice.

SUPPLEMENTARY DATA

Supplementary data related to this article can be found online at doi:10.1016/j.cvex. 2012.06.011.

REFERENCES

1. Heidenreich B. Pick a treat any treat. Good Bird Magazine 2008;4(4).
2. Sidman M. Coercion and its fallout. Boston: Authors Cooperative Inc., Publishers; 1989.
3. Heidenreich B. Understanding parrot body language. Austin, Texas: Good Bird Inc; 2008.
4. Husbandry RK. Animal training: successful animal management through positive reinforcement. Chicago: Shedd Aquarium Press; 1999.

Technicians and Exotic Animal Training

Alicea Schaeffer, BS, RVT, VTS (Behavior), KPA CTP

KEYWORDS

- Technicians • Behavioral history • Exotic animal behavior questions
- Husbandry training • Medical training • Behavioral classes
- Low-stress examination rooms • Behavioral enrichment

KEY POINTS

- Behavioral considerations are an essential element of patient care in veterinary hospitals.
- Medical training and low-stress examination rooms can be facilitated by veterinary technicians and are an important part of a veterinary visit.
- Technicians can play a vital role in client education, especially in behavioral education.
- Appropriate training and behavioral enrichment can contribute to animal health care.

INTRODUCTION

Technicians play a critical role in a veterinary practice. In many clinics the technician is responsible for collecting preliminary histories, drawing blood samples, placing intravenous catheters, administering and monitoring anesthesia, taking radiographs, client education, and so forth. The responsibilities of the technician are manifold. However, with a growing interest in addressing the behavioral and training needs of exotic patients, technicians have a new opportunity to enhance a practice's ability to serve its clients and patients. Technicians can be an important asset for the following:

- Collecting and documenting behavioral history of patients
- Providing low-stress handling during the veterinary examination
- Ensuring an animal's behavioral needs are met during the veterinary examination
- Meeting with clients and patients for nonexamination visits
- Teaching clients about training their animals for husbandry and cooperating in veterinary procedures
- Conducting classes on the basics of training with positive reinforcement

Hillview Veterinary Clinic, LLC, 1761 Thornburg Lane, Franklin, IN 46131, USA
E-mail address: alicearvt@yahoo.com

Vet Clin Exot Anim 15 (2012) 523–530
http://dx.doi.org/10.1016/j.cvex.2012.06.010
1094-9194/12/$ – see front matter © 2012 Elsevier Inc. All rights reserved.

vetexotic.theclinics.com

- Providing prepurchase counseling with an emphasis on preventing behavioral problems, early essential training, and behavioral expectations for different species
- Teaching clients about the benefits of enrichment and how to apply it

COLLECTING BEHAVIORAL HISTORY

A technician's responsibilities can include collecting a behavioral history on the patient. Depending on the species of animal, there are different questions to be addressed. Questions related to behavioral changes can reveal not only behavioral problems but also health problems long before the animal may show outward indicators of illness. It is important for the technician to keep detailed notes to allow records to be compared from year to year. Technicians can advise clients of the recommendation that exotic patients undergo yearly evaluations by the veterinarian, thus giving veterinary professionals an opportunity to observe behavioral patterns throughout the life of the patient. Technicians can inform clients about the amount of time their animal should spend performing certain behaviors, allowing clients to be more aware of normal behavior patterns and be attentive to any changes. Technicians can encourage clients to spend a little time each week observing their animal's activity, and help them develop an ethogram specific to each animal in the home.

To make behavioral history collecting easier, exotic patients can be grouped into 3 main categories: birds, reptiles, and small mammals. For most exotic animal practices, birds will make up a large percentage of the patient base and will have more behavioral issues than any other group. Routine questions can cover vocalizations, foraging, grooming, and interactions with caregivers. Pscittacines spend 40% to 60% of their waking time foraging for food.[1] Clients who are providing full bowls of food daily may have reduced foraging time down to 0%. Technicians can provide suggestions and resources to help clients increase their birds' foraging activities to increase physical activity and mental stimulation. Parrot vocalizations generally represent 2% to 5% of their time.[1] Social interactions take up 10% to 40% of their waking time.[1] During questioning a technician may discover undesired attention-seeking vocalizations are occurring at a high rate, and also may discover that the parrot is receiving little or no social interaction. These aspects can open the door for discussions on ways to address vocalizing for attention and how to deliver social interaction appropriately and sufficiently to address this commonly observed problem. (For an example of a comprehensive ethogram on wild parrots see Ref.[2]) Questions pertaining to light cycles, diet composition and amount, access to perceived nest sites, mate-like bonds with humans or parrots, and sleeping patterns can also be helpful when evaluating parrot behavior.

Reptile species commonly kept as pets represent a diverse group. Questions to ask about behavior will vary based on the species. It is important to gather information on the physical activities of the patient and make a comparison with normal activities for the species. For example, if the patient is a Tokay gecko, does it climb? If the patient is a green iguana, does its enclosure include branches suitable for climbing and does the animal make use of them? If the patient is a rock iguana or sand boa, does its enclosure include places to hide and/or a substrate suitable for burrowing? If the appropriate furnishings and substrate are available to the animal, one may ask if it actually uses them in a manner appropriate for that species. Behavioral questions can also cover social behavior including aggressive behavior toward the caregiver, other species of pets, and conspecifics. Technicians can also collect data on the amount of time spent basking and the type of light available (natural sunlight or artificial). Additional questions to ask include how often reptiles have access to water for soaking and how frequently the animal engages in this activity. It is also important to gather information on feeding practices including how food is presented, and the frequency and types of food offered. Having owners bring in photos of the animal's enclosure can assist technicians in evaluating whether the behavioral and enrichment needs of the animal are being met.

Small mammals also make up a large and diverse group. The following represents questions typically asked of clients with small exotic mammals. Some of these questions are also useful for avian and reptile patients. Additional questions for specific groups are listed also.

General questions for small mammals

- Does the animal have access to a conspecific?
- Describe the animal's social interactions with conspecifics.
- Describe the animal's social interactions with people.
- Describe aggressive behavior and the circumstances in which it might be presented.
- Describe fear or avoidance behaviors and the circumstances in which they might be presented.
- How much time does the animal spend outside of its enclosure? Supervised and unsupervised?
- Does the animal have access to places to hide, tunnel, or burrow?
- How much time does the animal spend interacting with toys or other enrichment items?
- Does the animal have foraging opportunities and does it engage in foraging activities?

Additional questions about ferret behavior

- Is the animal litter box trained?

Additional questions about rabbit behavior

- Is the animal litter box trained?
- Does the animal jump to/access perching areas such as an elevated platform, chair, and so forth?
- Does the animal engage in digging behaviors? If so, where and when?
- Does the animal have the opportunity to chew and shred enrichment items? How frequently are new chewable/shreddable items offered?

Additional questions about "pocket pets" (hamsters, gerbils, rats, mice)

- Does the animal engage in nest building activities? If so, for how long per day?
- Does the animal engage in digging behaviors? If so, where and when?
- Does the animal stow or cache food?
- Does the animal have an exercise wheel or other activity device and does it use it? If so, for how long per day?
- Does the animal have the opportunity to chew and shred enrichment items? How frequently are new chewable/shreddable items offered?

LOW-STRESS EXAMINATIONS

A veterinary professional's first priority is always the patient. In medicine it is important to "first, do no harm." When animals are unnecessarily overhandled in the veterinary hospital, it increases stress thereby causing potential harm. Low-stress restraint and handling has become an increasingly important objective for many practices. It is even more important for small exotic patients that can be easily stressed by handling. It is important for technicians to facilitate an examination so that the process is as hands-free as possible and includes minimal restraint procedures.

Technicians can also be available for patient visits to the clinic that do not involve medical care. Technicians can teach clients how to train their pets to voluntarily enter carriers and tolerate transport for a visit to the veterinary clinic. These visits are ideally done in the examination room and should involve at least one employee. The animal can be given the opportunity to come out of the carrier and receive preferred food items from its caregiver and staff members. Initially the animal may not accept the food or may prefer to stay in its transport container. Sometimes the first few visits will involve bringing the carrier into the examination room, opening the carrier, giving a food item, and the client and patient returning home.

There are additional ways technicians can help create a low-stress veterinary visit, one of which is to modify the examination room environment to address the needs of the exotic species scheduled for the appointment. For example, many exotic mammals and reptiles are highly sensitive to scents. Technicians can make sure that lingering odors of previous patients are eliminated. Another way to avoid stress is for technicians to be aware of the scheduling. Many practices see dogs and cats in addition to exotic animals. Technicians can review the schedule in advance to prepare for exotic animal appointments. Technicians can be prepared to move avian and small mammal patients into an examination room immediately, to avoid having to remain in a lobby that may include many dogs and cats. The preparations undertaken by a technician can help reduce or eliminate stress in exotic patients, thus improving not only the experience of the patient but also of the pet owner and veterinarian. If a patient is already showing indicators of stress before an examination begins, it may limit what the veterinarian will be able to accomplish and can affect blood chemistry values.

A technician's effort to replicate ideal conditions for an exotic animal will not go unnoticed by the pet owner or the patient. Small modifications that increase an animal's comfort can make a difference for the patient and also help foster good client relations. For example, if a reptile patient is scheduled, technicians can make sure the room is warm and that the examination table is not cold or at least covered to avoid direct contact with the cold surface. If it is cold outside, technicians can make sure the owner has equipped their carrier to keep the animal warm. Technicians can heat an examination glove full of tap water, wrap it in a towel, and set the reptile on it for a warmer ride home. If working with nocturnal animals, technicians can prepare the room by turning the lights down. Technicians can model behavior that facilitates keeping animals calm by moving slowly and talking softly around avian and exotic mammal patients.

HUSBANDRY AND MEDICAL TRAINING

Husbandry and medical training is most often used in zoos; however, it is gaining popularity in veterinary hospitals and with pet owners. This type of training focuses on teaching animals to cooperate in behaviors such as restraint, moving from one enclosure to another, delivery of medications, grooming, and so forth. Such conditioning is important because animals can become very stressed by some procedures, which might lead to further exacerbation of any existing health problems. For example, a parrot exhibiting pterotillomania (feather-damaging behaviors) may require daily medication. Involuntary capture and restraint of the bird followed by force feeding of oral medications may lead to increased stress responses, one of which may be increased feather-damaging behavior. Trying to hide medication in or on a preferred food item may also be inadequate, as it can result in an insufficient dose actually being ingested. Instead, training can be used to teach the bird to accept medications from a syringe, therefore avoiding stress and inadequate treatment.

Most animals at some point in their lives will require medications. Technicians can encourage clients to give their pets palatable fluids from syringes regularly so that when medications are needed there will be less stress and restraint. Ideally this is a behavior clients train before the animal becomes sick and needs medication. If this is not the case, training can still help the situation proceed more smoothly. For example, ferrets are generally receptive to the nutritional supplement called FerreTone. This supplement comes in a tube and can easily be drawn up into a syringe to be offered to a ferret. Once the ferret will accept the FerreTone from the syringe, the client can add a second syringe filled with medications. The ferret receives a small amount of FerreTone from the first syringe followed by some medication from the second syringe, which is then followed by more FerreTone. Another helpful training tool is to apply FerreTone to the outside of the medication syringe. This technique also works with rats and hamsters, using human baby food in place of FerreTone. Technicians who are responsible for medicating hospitalized patients can also use these techniques to deliver medications.

Targeting is another behavior technicians can easily train patients to present. (See the article by Heidenreich elsewhere in this issue for more information on targeting.) Target training has many hospital and home uses. Once the animal knows the behavior, technicians can use the target to direct an animal onto a scale, perch, or radiograph cassette, or into a cage. This hands-free method of moving an animal from place to place can greatly reduce stress as well as the risk of bites to staff members and clients.

There are many other behaviors that facilitate veterinary care that clients can easily teach their animals. Behaviors such as going into travel containers, accepting towels for restraint, toe-nail trims, and feather trims can all be trained using positive reinforcement at home. Teaching an animal to lay on its back and remain still is a useful behavior that aids in procedures such as taking radiographs, physical palpation, and blood draws. Technicians interested in and skilled at training with positive reinforcement can offer classes on animal training via the practice, thus giving clients additional assistance in accomplishing training goals for their exotic pets. This education also offers an additional product for practices to offer, and creates more opportunities for interaction with clients and their animals. Such interaction can help foster excellent client/practice relations as well as create patients that are cooperative in their own medical care.

BEHAVIOR CLASSES

Organized classes for pet owners are a huge benefit not only to the practice but also to the client. A monthly to bimonthly lecture on how animals learn can be offered at a small cost to clients. Because learning theory applies across all species, any owner with any species of animal will benefit. Teaching clients about operant and classical conditioning will help them understand why their animals perform certain behaviors and how they can increase or decrease these behaviors. Practices will want to make sure the training information provided is focused on positive reinforcement. Although other techniques based in the use of aversives are effective, it has been shown there is considerable fallout from the use of coercive training methods.[3] Technicians who teach behavior classes can educate clients about these undesired side effects of using aversives to train and encourage clients to avoid such techniques.

In addition to the basic application of positive reinforcement training techniques, classes can also include reading and interpreting animal body language. Successful animal training requires a good knowledge of when an animal is showing a fear response or aggressive behaviors, or appears calm and relaxed. Many bird owners report "their bird bites without warning." Although some birds do learn to mask body language associated with aggressive behavior, it is possible the client is not recognizing the precursors to aggressive behavior and is continuing with activities that lead to an escalation of aggressive responses (such as lunging and biting). Technicians can help clients learn to recognize the small changes in feather placement and body position; they can help clients be more observant and change their responses to help avoid a situation that might result in a bite. Teaching clients to be well versed in body language is also helpful to the technician when collecting behavioral histories. Educated clients will be better able to describe their pet's behavior. Classes also offer an opportunity for technicians to educate pet owners on normal and abnormal behavior for different exotic species, which can help clients know when something is wrong with their pet.

Unfortunately there is a lot of animal training information that can be dangerous for animals and clients. Clients may not always be able to distinguish good trainers from bad ones. Having a trusted source at their veterinary practice that is focused on the least intrusive, most positive science-based training technology is important. It can be the responsibility of a qualified veterinary technician to ensure clients receive good training information and also the skills necessary to train.

Offering training classes that involve clients' exotic pets can at times be difficult, because many exotic patients are not comfortable outside of the home environment. Bringing an exotic animal to a class may result in fear responses, which can make training a challenge. However, this is not impossible to overcome and can be a topic of study for the class. For those individuals that are comfortable in new environments it would be ideal to offer classes targeted toward each individual species, including rabbit-focused classes, ferret-focused classes, parrot-focused classes, and so forth. Clients and their animals are thus able to gather for classes and hands-on training opportunities. For clients attending without animals, animals can be provided for training or clients can practice training techniques on each other. All classes can focus on the practical application of positive-reinforcement training techniques and learning theory.

PREPURCHASING COUNSELING

Behavior problems are among the top reasons a pet is relinquished to an animal shelter.[4,5] Technicians can offer prepurchasing counseling to help prospective pet owners find the right pet. Technicians can ask questions about how much time the owner will have to interact and train the animal to help narrow down the selection. Technicians can help families with younger children to understand the social needs and responsibilities of caring for different types of pets. For example, if a child will only be able to interact with the pet in the afternoons, it might be suggested the family avoids a nocturnal animal such as a hedgehog and focuses on a guinea pig or ferret instead. Many prospective owners do not realize how long some birds and reptiles can live. Technicians can help clients understand what to expect behaviorally from different species of exotic animals commonly kept as pets. Such advice can help increase the likelihood that clients make informed decisions when acquiring an exotic pet.

BEHAVIORAL ENRICHMENT

The freedom to express normal behavior is included in the Five Freedoms presented by the Brambell Report (**Box 1**).[4]

Caregivers are often challenged to find ways to allow their animals to express normal behavior. Behavioral enrichment offers a solution to this dilemma. This aspect

---

Box 1
The Five Freedoms

- Freedom from hunger and thirst
- Freedom from discomfort
- Freedom from pain, injury, or disease
- Freedom to express normal behavior
- Freedom from fear and distress

---

of animal care is growing in popularity in zoos and aquariums, and also with dog trainers and small animal owners. Technicians have an opportunity to help clients learn about this important contribution to the quality of their exotic pet's life. "Enrichment should be positive, productive, interesting, and challenging, and a stimulation pursuit for animals that is rooted in 'natural' behavior."[6] To successfully provide enrichment, clients need to know their animal's natural history and personal history. Many animals that have never encountered enrichment devices may not know how to interact with them or may show a fear response. Some animals may need to be trained to interact with enrichment items. Technicians can help clients work through the approximations to teach an animal how to engage with enrichment devices. Technicians will also want to teach clients that if an animal responds favorably to enrichment items, these items can also function as reinforcers for behavior; this means clients will need to be taught that enrichment items can influence behavior. Timing of the delivery of enrichment will be important for clients to note. For example, if the client offers a parrot a toy to shred when it is vocalizing for attention, the appearance of a person and a desired toy could lead to an increase in undesired vocalizations. A technician could advise a client to offer the parrot the toy just before leaving the room when the bird is quiet, to engage the bird in acceptable activities, thus helping the bird be less inclined to vocalize when the preferred person leaves the room.

Training can also be enriching for animals. Technicians can help clients create training goals and shaping plans for each behavioral goal. Behaviors can include entertaining "tricks" such as turn around, lift a foot, or interact with props. These often easy-to-train behaviors can help clients learn about training. Successfully training a few simple behaviors can help motivate clients to keep adding behavior goals such as those helpful to medical care.

SUMMARY

Training and behavior are becoming increasingly popular areas of interest for pet owners. Clients need a trusted source for quality information on animal training that is based on science and noncoercive methods. The combination of addressing medical and behavioral needs of exotic animals allows a veterinary practice to provide added value for their clients. Technicians can play an important role in executing many aspects of a successful behavior program in a practice. From practical application in the examination room for hospitalized patients, to helping clients successfully train their animals at home, the end result is a cooperative patient and satisfied client.

REFERENCES

1. Bays T, Lightfoot T, Mayer J. Exotic pet behavior: birds, reptiles and small mammals. St Louis (MI): Saunders Elsevier; 2006. p. 53.

2. Snyder N, Wiley J, Kepler C. The parrots of Luquillo: natural history and conservation of the Puerto Rican parrot. Los Angeles (CA): Western Foundation of Vertebrate Zoology; 1987.

3. Sidman M. Coercion and its fallout. Boston: Authors Cooperative Inc; 1989. p. 80, 119, 186.

4. Scarlett J, Salman M, New J, et al. Reasons for relinquishment of companion animals in U.S. animal shelters: selected health and personal issues. J Appl Anim Welf Sci 1999;2:41–57.

5. Grandin T, Johnson C. Animals make us human: creating the best life for animals. New York: Houghton-Mifflin Harcourt; 2009.

6. Laule G, Ramirez K. Animal training; successful animal management through positive reinforcement. Chicago: Shedd Aquarium; 1999. p. 268.

Index

Note: Page numbers of article titles are in **boldface** type.

A

Vet Clin Exot Anim 15 (2012) 531–555
http://dx.doi.org/10.1016/S1094-9194(12)00070-9
1094-9194/12/$ – see front matter © 2012 Elsevier Inc. All rights reserved.

Moving?

Make sure your subscription moves with you!

To notify us of your new address, find your **Clinics Account Number** (located on your mailing label above your name), and contact customer service at:

Email: journalscustomerservice-usa@elsevier.com

800-654-2452 (subscribers in the U.S. & Canada)
314-447-8871 (subscribers outside of the U.S. & Canada)

Fax number: 314-447-8029

Elsevier Health Sciences Division
Subscription Customer Service
3251 Riverport Lane
Maryland Heights, MO 63043

*To ensure uninterrupted delivery of your subscription, please notify us at least 4 weeks in advance of move.

Printed and bound by CPI Group (UK) Ltd, Croydon, CR0 4YY

03/10/2024

01040439-0019